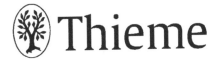

An Approach to Successful Stapedectomy

B. M. Gupta, MS (ENT), DLO
Senior Otologist
Gupta ENT Hospital
Nagpur, Maharashtra, India

Thieme
Delhi • Stuttgart • New York • Rio de Janeiro

Publishing Director: Ritu Sharma
Development Editor: Dr Gurvinder Kaur
Director-Editorial Services: Rachna Sinha
Project Manager: Madhumita Dey
Vice President, Sales and Marketing: Arun Kumar Majji
Managing Director & CEO: Ajit Kohli

Thieme Medical and Scientific Publishers Private Limited.
A - 12, Second Floor, Sector - 2, Noida - 201 301,
Uttar Pradesh, India, +911204556600
Email: customerservice@thieme.in
www.thieme.in

Cover design: © Thieme
Cover image source: © Thieme

Page make-up by RECTO Graphics, India

Printed in India

5 4 3 2

ISBN: 978-93-90553-10-5
eISBN: 978-93-90553-18-1

Contents

Preface

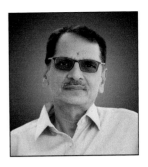

Stapedectomy is the only surgery in otology where the results are immediate, however it is the most delicate surgery too.

I have been performing this surgery for more than 3.5 decades. During this time I operated on a large number of patients. I came across several difficult situations and a variety of problems during the surgeries. Fortunately, I could handle most of them successfully.

During the initial years of my practice, I had only picks and perforators, as there was no microdrill at that time. Later, I acquired the microdrill that helped me handle difficult situations with more ease and confidence.

Addition of a CO_2 laser in my instruments list was a big landmark. Although, the instrument was very expensive, but it immensely helped me in handling such a delicate bone atraumatically, to avoid complications during surgery, and to get good hearing results. Lasers are very useful not only for primary surgery but also for revision surgery. The use of laser in stapes surgery has improved the hearing results, with lesser chances of vertigo after surgery, hence shorter hospital stay.

It is also to be kept in mind that very young patients with conductive hearing loss with normal tympanic membrane are not necessarily patients of otosclerosis. The possibility of congenital ossicular anomaly and facial nerve anomaly should always be considered and should be investigated accordingly before surgery.

This book documents various surgeries including all the difficult situations encountered by me during my practice. It also comprises a series of photographs showing each and every step of surgery to aid easy understanding of the subject. This makes the book unique and different from other books.

I am very sure this book will guide the junior otologist friends and will help in making them better stapes surgeons.

Before I end, I would like to thank my wife, Dr Mrs Vijaylaxmi Gupta and my daughters, Sheetal and Dr Sneha for helping me in writing this book.

B. M. Gupta, MS (ENT), DLO
Senior Otologist
Gupta ENT Hospital
Nagpur, Maharashtra, India

1 Introduction

There are very few occasions that an ear, nose, and throat (ENT) surgeon cherishes the most. A successful stapedectomy is one of them. When the surgery is performed under local anesthesia, the pleasure of sudden improvement in the hearing after putting the piston during surgery is the moment that is cherished the most, by both the patient and the surgeon.

Hearing improvement in stapedectomy is far more superior to that in tympanoplasty, with minimum or no complications if proper care is taken while selecting the case and if proper technique is used during surgery.

Stapedectomy is a surgery that otherwise looks simple, but it is not, as there are a lot of difficult situations that are faced by an experienced surgeon while doing many cases, which makes him more cautious while performing each and every case.

Stapedectomy is the most technical and demanding surgery and there are a lot of expectations from the surgeon. These expectations of the patient are to be fulfilled by doing a perfect job. During surgery when everything goes right and perfect, you will end up with a happy patient with good hearing and a satisfied surgeon.

If something goes wrong, you will end up with a dizzy and frightened patient. This dizziness takes a lot of time to settle down with decreased hearing or no hearing, which is irreversible (lifetime trouble). This means that there is a very narrow margin between success and failure.

Therefore, a stapedectomy surgeon has to do a perfect job to achieve stable and long-term hearing results, so his basic ideas should be clear and he should be competent enough to handle all the possible situations.

The aim of writing this book is to present recent innovations and current scientific concepts in stapes surgery. The aim is to make surgery safe and atraumatic and to give good long-term hearing results after surgery. Remember that there is no chance of RE-DO in stapes surgery unlike other middle ear surgeries. Hence, the first surgical effort should be the best effort.

2 History of Stapedectomy

The following points list the milestones achieved by stapedectomy:

- In 1893, Politzer was the first person to describe stapes fixation.

- After that, attempts were made by various surgeons to mobilize the stapes or to remove the stapes, but at that time, the ossicular chain was not reconstructed. All surgeries failed due to infection and temporary hearing improvement.

- After a long gap, in 1941, it was Lempert who performed the fenestration operation to improve hearing without causing sensorineural hearing loss.

- In 1953, Rosen while performing some other middle ear surgical procedure accidentally mobilized the stapes of a deaf patient under local anesthesia, and the patient was very much delighted with the sudden improvement in the hearing.

- In 1956, John Shea performed the first stapedectomy and he kept a piece of bone between the oval window and the incus. There was an immediate improvement in the hearing, which deteriorated afterward, which could be due to some technical error.

- In 1960 John Shea placed a teflon piston attached it to long process of incus and other end was placed in to the hole made in the stapes footplate. This was the first successful stapedectomy.

- In 1960, Schuknecht used fat wire prosthesis, in which fat is used to cover the footplate fenestra and a wire attached to the fat was used for reconstruction of the ossicular chain.

- After that, various innovations have taken place in stapes surgery. Earlier it was a large fenestra surgery (stapedectomy). Later on, it is small fenestra surgery (stapedotomy).

- Earlier 0.5- or 0.6-mm-thick Teflon pistons were used. Now 0.4-mm-thick pistons are placed in a 0.6-mm fenestra. Recently, titanium prostheses of various types are being used by many surgeons.

- Earlier the tissue seal used at the fenestra was connective tissue. Later on, Causse started the vein graft interposition technique.

- Earlier surgery was performed using various picks and perforators. Later on, microdrills were used, which made the surgery safer. Now with CO_2 laser, surgery has become very much atraumatic with minimal or no complication.

3 Expected Difficulties during Stapes Surgery

When one plans for a stapedectomy, some difficulties are expected. It may so happen that the surgeon may encounter some difficult situation that he never expected. The surgeon should be prepared to handle this difficult situation. Surgeons should be armed with necessary instruments to handle the following situations:

- First and foremost, diagnosis should be correct and surgery should be performed in the right patient. Special attention is to be paid for unilateral sensorineural hearing loss with false-negative Rinne. Here the Weber test will be toward the normal ear.

- Narrow canal wall and bulging anterior and posterior bony canal wall may require endaural incision with canaloplasty.

- At times, meatal skin is very thin and delicate with the possibility of tear if care is not taken.

- There may be a patient with big bony overhang almost hiding the stapes completely. In such patient lot of overhang removal is required.

- Very narrow oval window slit with very deep and hidden footplate of the stapes.

- Dehiscent facial nerve, at times complete, may hide the footplate.

- Various congenital anomalies like abnormal facial nerve, short or malformed incus, malleus head fixation, persistent stapedial artery, and other ossicular anomalies may be seen.

Management of these situations is discussed later on in subsequent chapters.

4 Otosclerosis: Clinical Histopathology

Otosclerosis occurs only in the temporal bone. Otosclerosis is a disease affecting only the otic capsule involving only the stapes and not affecting the malleus and the incus. No other bones in the body are involved. It is a localized disorder of bone metabolism of the otic capsule in which matured lamellar bone is replaced by spongy, thicker, highly cellular, and vascular bone.

There are three varieties:

1. Stapedial: This causes conductive deafness due to involvement of the stapes, its footplate, and oval window.

2. Cochlear: This causes purely sensorineural hearing loss due to the involvement of the cochlear endosteum, which is rare.

3. Combined: Most of the time, the disease is combined, with stapedial and cochlear pathology both causing a mixed variety of deafness. This is the commonest among all.

One more entity described is histological otosclerosis, where the disease does not manifest clinically, but there are otosclerotic foci here and there in the temporal bone not affecting stapedial and cochlear function. The patient remains asymptomatic throughout his life.

Otosclerotic focus causing stapedial fixation can lead to air–bone (AB) gap of up to 60 db. In early otosclerosis, bony fixation of anterior footplate causes an AB gap of up to 30 to 40 dB. Diffuse otosclerosis due to involvement of the entire circumference of the annular ligament result in conductive hearing loss of 50 dB, but the degree of footplate fixation cannot be predicted by the AB gap in all the cases. Minimal footplate fixation is often found in cases with large AB gaps. In minimal footplate fixation, the risk of getting floating footplate is very high. Hence, a floater can even occur in patients with large AB gaps. Otosclerosis focus can involve any part of the otic capsule but few common sites causing conductive or mixed variety of deafness are the following:

- Anterior to the oval window.

- Posterior to the oval window.

- Circumferential involvement of the footplate.

- Biscuit type (thick) footplate.

- Obliterative.

- Round window involvement.

Among all foci, anterior to the oval window focus is commonest. The second most common site is involvement of the round window area, but total obliteration of the round window is rare. Round window obliteration is associated with conductive hearing loss. Another common site involving the otosclerotic focus is posterior to the oval window. Other uncommon sites are the internal auditory meatus, near the cochlear aqueduct, and the semicircular canal. The disease is usually bilateral in 70 to 80% of cases.

5 Clinical Aspect of Otosclerosis

Introduction

Deafness in otosclerosis is gradually progressive. It is usually bilateral symmetrical or asymmetrical. Generally, it affects the second, third, and fourth decades of life (most active part of life) and it is more common in females than in males. Family history of deafness is present most of the time. In females, it is aggravated during pregnancy.

Diagnosis

- History is very much diagnostic. Along with the deafness, patient's voice is very typical. They speak very softly as they hear their own voice loudly in the affected ears.

- Clinical examination is normal. Tympanic membrane is normal.

- Tuning fork test is the most reliable test and is very much diagnostic.

- Rinne's test is negative.

- Weber's test is toward the worse ear.

- False-negative Rinne tests should always be kept in mind in unilateral sensorineural hearing loss (SNHL). Here the weber test will be toward the opposite ear (better ear).

- One rare possibility of a third mobile window, especially superior semicircular canal dehiscence, should always be kept in mind.

If there is no improvement in hearing following surgery and there is no closure of air–bone (AB) gap following stapedectomy, a third mobile window should be suspected after ruling out other causes of persistent conductive hearing loss following stapedectomy.

- Audiometry: Pure tone audiogram (PTA) shows conductive hearing loss or mixed hearing loss with an AB gap (**Fig. 5.1a, b**). The Carhart notch (a drop in the bone conduction at 1,000–2,000 Hz) is present in most of the patients, which disappears after successful surgery.

- The hearing loss in early fixation of footplate is for low frequency, but as the disease advances, all the frequencies are involved.

- Impedance audiogram is done to confirm the diagnosis and to rule out any fluid in the middle ear.

In otosclerosis, there is normal middle ear pressure, low compliance in tympanometry (as pattern), and absent acoustic reflex (**Fig. 5.1c**).

Acoustic reflex is absent in patients with otosclerosis but present in cases of third mobile window in which there is also an AB gap. Hence, acoustic reflex should always be done in patients of conductive hearing loss.

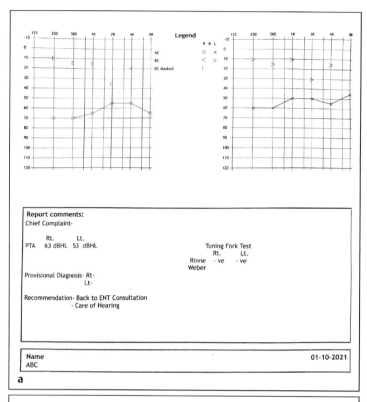

Fig. 5.1 Pure tone audiogram. **(a)** Bilateral mixed hearing loss with a 45- to 50-dD air–bone (AB) gap with the Carhart notch at 2000 Hz. **(b)** Mixed hearing loss in the right ear with a 40-db AB gap with the Carhart notch at 2,000 Hz. *(Continued)*

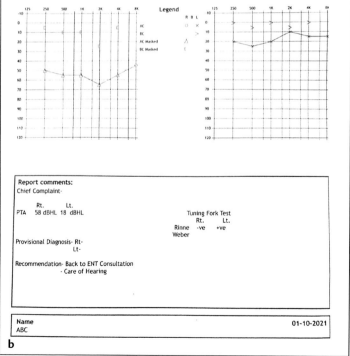

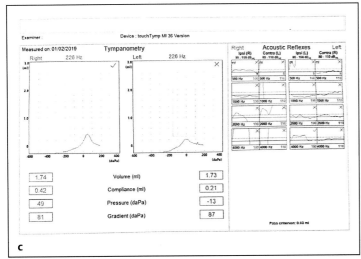

Fig. 5.1 *(Continued)* Pure tone audiogram. **(c)** Impedance audiogram: low compliance in tympanometry (As pattern, normal middle ear pressure, absent acoustic reflex in both the ears).

Various audiological tests are available, but the tuning fork test remains the most dependable test. It is a quick and reliable way of assessing the type and nature of hearing loss. The results of PTA and impedance audiometry are to be matched with tuning fork tests. The results of the audiometry test done at various centers may vary and when there is some confusion, surgeons should rely more on the tuning fork test than on any other test.

6 Imaging before Stapedectomy

Diagnosing otosclerosis clinically is not difficult. History, clinical examination, tuning fork test, and audiogram confirm the diagnosis.

Routinely high-resolution computed tomography (HRCT) scan of the temporal bone is not done in India as it is not required in all the cases. Cost factor also plays a very important role.

CT scan of the temporal bone should always be done in very young patients (the 10- to 20-year age group) reporting with conductive or mixed hearing loss with normal tympanic membrane, with or without facial deformity. This is done to confirm the diagnosis and to find out any congenital anomalies in the middle ear like anomalies of facial nerve and ossicles. Abnormally wide cochlear aqueduct, if found during CT scan, warns the operating surgeon with the possibility of perilymph gusher; hence, HRCT temporal bone should be done when congenital footplate fixation is suspected.

When the disease is active, decalcification takes place at the margins of the oval window. Hence, the oval window looks bigger than normal. When there is sclerosis, there is new bone formation, and the oval window looks narrow. In obliterative otosclerosis, the oval window is obliterated. Hence, CT scan of the temporal bone helps in getting an idea about the activity and extent of the disease.

CT scan of the temporal bone should always be done in patients with sensorineural hearing loss (SNHL) to confirm cochlear otosclerosis and far advanced otosclerosis.

Double ring effect due to multiple active foci coming together or mosaic effect due to alternate active or inactive foci helps in diagnosis, along with history and clinical examination. In far advanced otosclerosis, if cochlear implant is planned, cochlear lumen should always be confirmed by either CT scan or magnetic resonance imaging (MRI).

CT scan of the temporal bone should be done in patients of otosclerosis having vertigo to know any other pathology responsible for vertigo. CT scan temporal bone also help to rule out other causes of conductive hearing loss with normal ear drum like ossicular discontinuity.

Rare conditions like round window obliteration and dehiscent superior semicircular canal can also be ruled out by CT scan of the temporal bone. In these conditions, hearing loss may be conductive or of a mixed variety.

Before revision surgery, HRCT of the temporal bone gives a lot of useful information. If the patient has developed sensorineural hearing loss after the first surgery associated with vertigo, possibility of long piston and perilymph fistula should be ruled out. In perilymph fistula, pneumolabyrinth may be seen even after 3 weeks after surgery.

Short piston, erosion of the long process of the incus, and displacement of the prosthesis presenting as conductive hearing loss, long after first the surgery, can also be diagnosed. Displaced prosthesis deep into the vestibule can be detected, which is associated with vertigo and SNHL. Both Teflon and titanium prosthesis can be visualized in CT scan, but both have variable hyperdensities in CT scan.

Hence, HRCT of the temporal bone done before a revision surgery gives a lot of useful information, and various difficult situations are diagnosed before planning for surgery so that surgeons can handle these situations comfortably. In addition, HRCT of the temporal bone should be done when surgery in the second ear is planned.

Cone beam CT scan is superior to routine multidetector CT (MDCT) scan, as there is minimal radiation and better visualization. Fine cuts (slice thickness of 0.5 mm) are required for complete visualization.

7 Surgical Treatment of Otosclerosis

Most of the cases of stapedial otosclerosis are suitable for stapes surgery. There should be an adequate air–bone gap and good cochlear reserve for successful outcome. Conductive deafness of more than 20 dB with a negative Rinne test, with normal tympanic membrane, is an indication for stapedectomy.

When the disease is bilateral, the poor hearing ear is selected first.

If the air–bone gap is less than 20 dB, it means the disease is at an early stage and there is minimal footplate fixation. It is always better to wait for the surgery as there is a risk of getting a floating footplate with early fixation; however, the scenario has changed now since CO_2 laser is used for stapedotomy. These early cases can also be operated on now with CO_2 laser, as the surgery is very much atraumatic with CO_2 laser without any risk and complication.

In combined otosclerosis, surgery should always be done if there is good air–bone gap and there is a good cochlear reserve with good speech discrimination.

Regarding the age of the patient, there is no upper limit if the patient is fit for surgery. Patients up to the age of 90 years can be operated on with satisfactory results if cochlear reserve is good and there is good speech discrimination score. For very young patients, the possibility of congenital middle ear and inner ear anomalies should be kept especially when there is mixed hearing loss. High-resolution computed tomography (HRCT) scan of the temporal bone should be done specially to detect any inner ear abnormalities. The possibility of obliterative otosclerosis is very high in young patients.

At times, the disease is unilateral, with the other ear having a normal hearing. These patients should always be operated on to get equal, symmetrical hearing in both ears, which is very much useful for localization of sound.

8 | Innovation in Stapes Surgery

Introduction

Revolution leads to innovation. New ideas are generated and converted into useful technology. Many innovations have taken place in stapes surgery like surgical instruments, surgical techniques, and prosthesis used.

Various innovations that have taken place in stapes surgery in the last few years are briefly explained in this chapter.

Stapedectomy to Stapedotomy

Earlier it was total removal of the footplate, then partial removal, and now it is a small fenestra surgery.

Earlier it was stapedectomy with a teflon piston of 0.6 mm. Now it is stapedotomy of 0.6 mm with a Teflon piston of 0.4 mm.

Titanium prosthesis is also used in place of a teflon piston.

Seal around the Piston at the Fenestra

Earlier it was connective tissue seal or no seal at the fenestra.

Now people are practicing the vein graft interposition technique, which is very safe.

Blood clot as tissue seal is also used by many people. Clotted blood is made up of fibrin, which acts as a stronger tissue seal.

No statistically increased incidence of sensorineural hearing loss (SNHL) following surgery is observed when no tissue seal is placed as compared to cases with tissue seal.

Instruments Used

Earlier picks and perforators were used for surgery. Now microdrills are used in addition to them. Laser is the latest addition to the surgical tool for stapedotomy.

The conventional technique of stapes surgery by using picks and perforators is crude and risky. Microdrills have made stapedectomy safe and simple.

CO_2 laser has made surgery very much atraumatic and safe. Very difficult situations can be handled by the surgeon, making him more confident, thus improving the results of surgery.

9 Contraindications for Surgery

Introduction

Most of the contraindications for stapedectomy are relative and surgery can be performed in these cases once the patient is made fit for surgery. There is only one absolute contraindication for stapedectomy, which is discussed in the following section.

Absolute Contraindications

Surgery should not be done in the **only hearing ear** as there is around 1 to 2% risk of getting total sensorineural hearing loss following surgery, which may be early or late.

These patients should be given hearing aid. In the only hearing ear with advanced disease where the conventional hearing aid is not very useful, a bone-anchored hearing aid (BAHA) is a very good alternative. The main advantage of using a BAHA is that there is no risk of dead ear following insertion of a BAHA, which is very much there with stapedectomy. In addition, the sound quality with a BAHA is better than the conventional hearing aid.

Relative Contraindications

- Upper respiratory infection (URI) with eustachian tube (ET) block and external ear and middle ear infection: In such cases, treat the condition and then perform the surgery. The external auditory canal should also be free from infection and exostoses. If exostosis is found, it should be treated first and then stapedectomy is performed once the canal is completely healed and epithelialized.

- In patients with general medical disease like uncontrolled diabetes and hypertension, control the disease and then perform the surgery.

- Otosclerosis with hydrops: Otosclerosis associated with endolymphatic hydrops is not uncommon. Deafness is associated with vertigo, which at times is severe. Vertigo should be controlled before surgery. Patients should have a minimum of 6 months of vertigo-free period before the surgery.

- Positive Schwartz sign: It is present at times especially in young patients, which indicates that the disease is very active. These cases should be treated by fluorides before surgery. Sodium fluoride with calcium is given to these patients for 6 to 12 months. This reduces the activity of otosclerotic focus and surgery can be performed comfortably.

- During pregnancy: Focus is active during pregnancy and after. Hence, a 6-month gap after delivery should always be there. During this phase, the otosclerotic focus becomes less active and silent. Then surgery can be performed without any hurdle.

- In patients who are involved in vigorous physical activity like wrestling and boxing, stapedectomy should be postponed till they give up these activities. Similarly, skydivers and scuba divers are at risk of barotrauma following stapedectomy if the ET function is compromised.

10 Preoperative Counseling

All the patients should be told about the disease process. They should be explained where and what exactly is involved in this disease, and surgical procedures should always be properly explained to them in their language. They should always be told about the rare possibility of getting permanent hearing loss after surgery, an incidence that has now become very less with the use of laser in this surgery.

They should be told regarding alternative measures like hearing aid.

They should also be informed about the postoperative precautions if surgery is done.

Patients who are involved with flying, scuba diving, and parachuting are more prone to barotrauma following a stapes surgery. They should be warned regarding the possibility of irreversible damage, and these activities should be avoided after stapedectomy especially when associated with poor eustachian tube (ET) function. Certain centers allow these activities after confirming the ET function by performing a tympanometry.

11 Otosclerosis and Vertigo

Patients with otosclerosis may present with positional vertigo, which is usually minor and is not a contraindication for surgery.

Certain patients suffer from severe degree of episodic vertigo with sensorineural hearing loss (SNHL; mixed hearing loss) due to associated endolymphatic hydrops. This is the contraindication for surgery as the dilated saccule in endolymphatic hydrops lies very close to the stapedial footplate and may get traumatized while making the fenestra. These hydrops should always be controlled by giving betahistine (vertin) for a long time, and a 6-month symptom-free period is necessary before surgery. Otoflour may also be required along with Betahistine to cool down the disease.

It was found recently that the saccule does not come close to the footplate in the cases where the preoperative bone conduction was less than 35 db at a frequency of 500 Hz, and there was no high-frequency hearing loss. Surgery in these cases was reported to be successful.

12 Otosclerosis with Tinnitus

Most of the causes of tinnitus are untreatable. In otosclerosis along with deafness, tinnitus is not an uncommon complaint. The tinnitus in otosclerosis comes in the category of treatable cause of tinnitus. The exact cause of tinnitus is not known and it is found mostly in patients with combined otosclerosis having sensorineural components. Some vascular or enzymatic factor is said to be responsible for tinnitus and this tinnitus may increase as the disease progresses. Tinnitus is not a contraindication for surgery and may disappear after surgery in 70% of patients. In the remaining patients, tinnitus remains the same after surgery and in around 5% of patients, tinnitus may increase after surgery. This should always be explained to the patient before surgery and informed consent should always be taken before surgery. Tinnitus is said to be decreased by giving Otoflour for a long time, and this should always be started before surgery along with calcium.

13 Instruments

Instruments used for stapes surgery are standard with little variations from person to person (**Fig. 13.1**). Most important instruments used for stapedectomy are the following:

- Speculum holders, which leave both the hands free, can be used. Routine practice in India is to hold the speculum with the left hand and perform the surgery with the right hand or vice versa.

- Good operating microscope with good illumination (Xenon or light-emitting diode [LED]) is necessary as it is mandatory to use higher magnification while working on the footplate, and you should be able to get good illumination while working with higher magnification for surgical precision and accuracy.

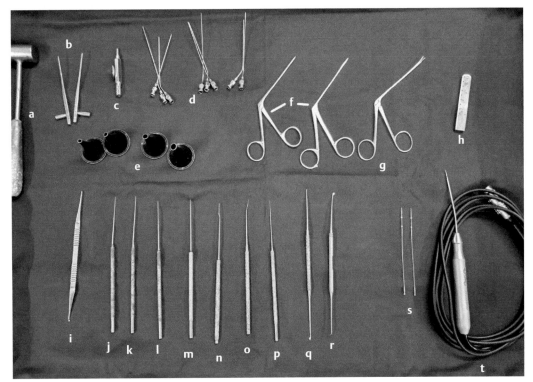

Fig. 13.1 Instruments used for stapedectomy are **(a)** hammer, **(b)** 1.00-mm gauge, **(c)** suction–adaptor, **(d)** suction cannulas, **(e)** set of ear speculum, **(f)** micro-forceps, **(g)** micro-scissors, **(h)** piston cutting jig, **(i)** double-ended curette, **(j–m)** straight and right angle pick, **(n)** piston measuring rod, **(o)** angled pick, **(p)** 0.4-mm disk, **(q, r)** side circular knife, and **(s, t)** Microdrill with bur.

14 Prosthesis

The prosthesis used for stapedectomy should be biocompatible, corrosion free, and should not cause any allergic reaction. Among various prosthesis available, Teflon and titanium pistons are the most popular and well-accepted prostheses used for stapedectomy.

The most commonly used pistons in India are Teflon pistons.

Teflon pistons of various thicknesses and lengths should be readily available in the trolley.

A 0.4-mm-thick piston is most commonly used. A 0.3-mm-thick piston is needed at times in a very narrow oval window niche. It should be available in your trolley (**Fig. 14.1**).

A Teflon piston with a narrow loop (0.63 mm) known as Shea's piston is required for a thin incus.

Malleus to stapes footplate piston should be available for malleostapedotomy.

Titanium Nitinol pistons are also used by a few surgeons, but they are costly.

Robinson bucket handle prosthesis is needed for a short incus. Here it is not possible to put a normal Teflon piston (**Fig. 14.2**). This should also be available in the trolley.

Earlier there was a trend of using large-diameter pistons, with the opinion that large-diameter piston leads to stronger transmission of sound energy, but large fenestra surgery is more traumatic than

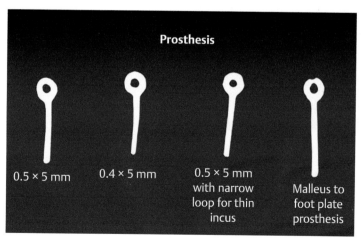

Prosthesis

0.5 × 5 mm   0.4 × 5 mm   0.5 × 5 mm with narrow loop for thin incus   Malleus to foot plate prosthesis

Fig. 14.1 Teflon pistons of various thickness and sizes should be readily available. A 0.3-mm-thick piston is needed in a very narrow oval window niche.

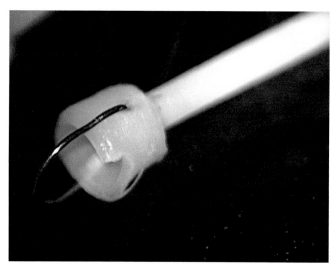

Fig. 14.2 Robinson bucket handle prosthesis, very useful for a short incus, used with vein graft interposition.

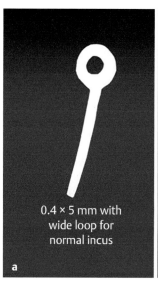 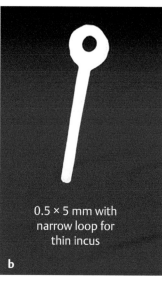

0.4 × 5 mm with wide loop for normal incus

a

0.5 × 5 mm with narrow loop for thin incus

b

Fig. 14.3 (a) A 0.4 × 5 mm Teflon piston with wide loop for a normal incus. (b) A 0.5 × 5 mm Teflon piston with narrow loop for a thin incus.

small fenestra surgery. Hence, ultimately, a 0.6-mm fenestra with a 0.4-mm piston is the standard (**Fig. 14.3**).

The weight of the prosthesis also plays a very big role in giving hearing results. Heavier pistons (metallic) may give better hearing results in the lower frequencies, and lighter pistons (Teflon) may give better hearing results in the higher frequencies.

Whichever prosthesis is used, the length of the prosthesis should be perfect, and it should not project more than 0.25 mm into the vestibule. The longer prosthesis could result in vestibular symptoms and shorter prosthesis could result in conductive deafness, and there is a high possibility of migration of prosthesis from oval window fenestra when prosthesis is short.

15 Anesthesia for Stapedotomy

Introduction

Stapedotomy can be performed under either local or general anesthesia.

Usually local anesthesia (2% Xylocaine with 1 in 2,00,000 adrenaline) with light sedation is preferred. Some antianxiety preparations should be given a night before the surgery. Light sedation during surgery gives a chance to test the hearing of the patient on the operation table immediately after inserting the piston. During surgery, if the patient complains of vertigo when the piston is inserted, it means that the piston is longer and corrective measures should be taken immediately. This is the advantage of local anesthesia.

Many surgeons prefer general anesthesia for this surgery as they feel that both the surgeon and the patient are comfortable with general anesthesia. In a very anxious and uncooperative patients, it is better to do surgery under general anesthesia. In general anesthesia, it is also necessary to do local infiltration with adrenaline to reduce bleeding.

Either of these anesthesia can be used for primary cases, as there is no difference in the final outcome with local or general anesthesia in primary cases. However, in revision surgeries, local anesthesia is always preferred, as the patient under local anesthesia with minimal sedation can complain immediately regarding the vertigo that he gets while manipulating the prosthesis at the footplate fenestra so that immediate action can be taken. Similar feedback is not possible under general anesthesia, and manipulation of the prosthesis at the footplate fenestra may damage the inner ear structure leading to sensorineural hearing loss.

Local Anesthesia Infiltration

The meatus is infiltrated at the 12, 3, 6, and 9 o'clock positions and 2 ml to 3 mL of 2% Xylocaine with adrenaline is sufficient (**Fig. 15.1**).

Infiltration should be done bone deep, just medial to the junction of the cartilaginous and bony meatus.

Avoid raising blebs while infiltrating. A bleb is formed if the infiltration is not done deep to the periosteum and if the quantity of infiltration is more (**Fig. 15.2**).

Slight infiltration at the opening of the external auditory meatus is done to avoid pain while pushing the biggest possible speculum into the external auditory canal.

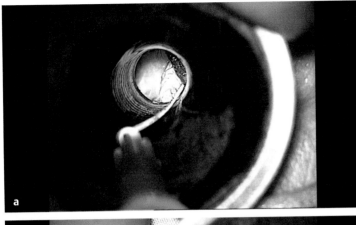

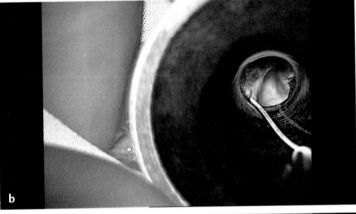

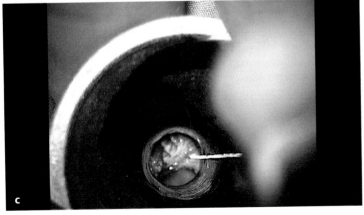

Fig. 15.1 Infiltration of the right ear meatus at the junction of the cartilaginous and bony meatus. **(a)** The meatus is infiltrated at the 6 o'clock position. **(b)** The meatus is infiltrared at the 9 o'clock position. **(c)** The meatus is infiltrated at the 3 o 'clock position. *(Continued)*

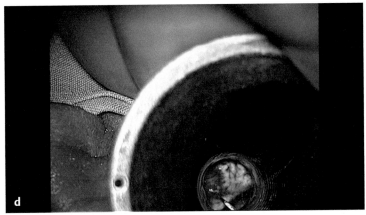

Fig. 15.1 *(Continued)* Infiltration of the right ear meatus at the junction of the cartilaginous and bony meatus. **(d)** The meatus is infiltrated at the 12 o'clock position.

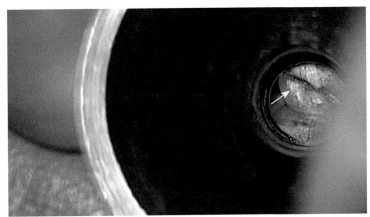

Fig. 15.2 Avoid raising blebs while infiltrating. The *arrow* shows bleb.

16 Incision

The endomeatal incision is the most common surgical approach. An endaural incision is required when the meatus is narrow. If the surgeon is not comfortable with the endomeatal incision, it is better to start the surgery with the endaural incision rather than struggling with the endomeatal incision. The endaural incision required here is very small, not the classical endaural incision, which is bigger (**Fig. 16.1**). Beginners should start their career with the endaural incision and then gradually shift to the endomeatal incision once they are confident.

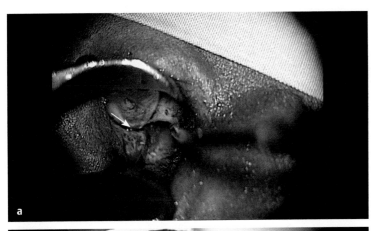

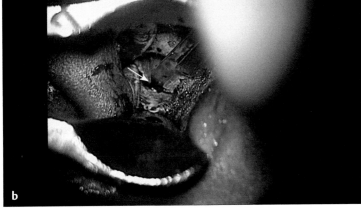

Fig. 16.1 **(a)** A small endaural incision, *arrow* (first vertical part) mostly within the canal. **(b)** A small endaural incision, *arrow* (second horizontal part). *(Continued)*

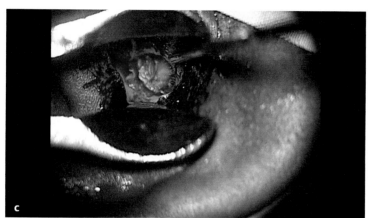

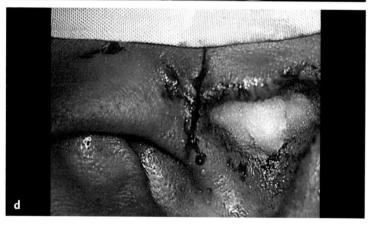

Fig. 16.1 *(Continued)* **(c)** A small endaural incision with adequate exposure. **(d)** A small endaural incision. One stitch is enough to close the incision.

17 Basic Principles of Stapes Surgery

Introduction

Before starting surgery, proper positioning of the head of the patient is very important. The head of the patient should be turned toward the other side with little extension of the neck by 10 degrees so that there is proper visualization of the stapes area. The operation table is adjusted so that the external auditory canal and the tympanic membrane are horizontal. All the steps in this surgery are equally important. Remember that for doing a perfect job, the surgeon should never be in a hurry.

A speculum holder is used by few surgeons, which keeps both the hands of the surgeon free.

An ear speculum of proper size is selected. If it is small, it restricts the view. If it is large, its tip pushes the soft tissue of the external auditory canal, especially the cartilaginous part, medially restricting the view.

Endomeatal incision is a curved incision starting from the 6 o'clock position going up to the 12 o'clock and should be around 1 cm from the sulcus at the 3 and 9 o'clock positions, in left and right ears, respectively. The tympanomeatal (TM) flap should be large enough to cover the posterosuperior bony meatal wall defect created after removal of the meatal wall overhang. The flap is elevated simultaneously from all the sides and the middle ear is entered just below the chorda tympani nerve. The TM flap is pushed forward and remains folded anteriorly.

Exposure to the middle ear is very important for easy working in the footplate area, especially in difficult situations. It is the key to success in this surgery.

The chorda tympani nerves should be preserved as much as possible.

For sufficient exposure, the posterosuperior bony meatal wall overhang is removed either by a curette or by a micro-drill with diamond bur. A 1-mm gauge with a hammer can also be used gently.

After removal of posterosuperior bony meatal wall overhang, surgeons should be able to see the neck of the malleus above and the round window below. Posteriorly, the base of the pyramid should be visible. Complete footplate of the stapes with the posterior crura should be visible.

Overexposure should be avoided. The body of the incus should not be exposed (**Fig. 17.1**).

Once you open the middle ear, check all the ossicles. Palpate all the ossicles separately, to see for their mobility. also, look for any malleus head fixation. Confirm the stapes fixation. All these assessments are again confirmed after disarticulating the incudostapedial (IS) joint. Once otosclerosis is confirmed, the surgeon can go ahead with stapedotomy. Before that, the round window should be examined for any otosclerotic focus, especially in the cases with extensive disease. Complete round window obliteration is rare.

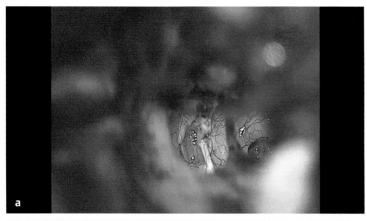

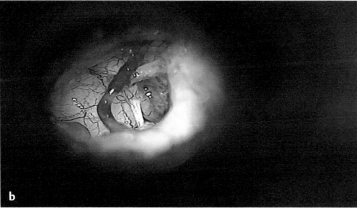

Fig. 17.1 (a) Exposure required during stapedectomy (right ear). (b) Exposure required during stapedectomy (left ear).

The footplate area should always be examined under higher magnification so that one can plan according to the type of footplate, which is either thin blue or thick and obliterative.

Mucosa over the footplate should always be decongested by keeping a gelfoam soaked in adrenaline for 7 minutes. The mucosa over the footplate area should be removed or the footplate is demucosalized so that the raw footplate bone is exposed before making the fenestra.

The next step is to cut the stapedius muscle by scissors or a sickle knife.

A fenestra of 0.6 mm is made in the posterior part of the footplate either by pick or perforator or by a microdrill. Earlier, it was suggested that the posterior part of the footplate is the safest area for making a fenestra, but now it is confirmed that it is the middle third of the footplate, especially its inferior part, which is the safest area for making a fenestra as the distance between the undersurface of footplate and the membranous labyrinth is maximum here. The fenestra can be made either before removal of the stapes superstructure or after removal of the stapes superstructure.

Posterior crura can be drilled by a micro-drill. The incudostapedial joint is separated by a right angle pick. The superstructure is removed by fracturing it toward the promontory by a right angle pick. The distance between the stapes footplate and the undersurface of the incus is measured by distance measuring rods and to it 0.25 mm is added for the thickness of the footplate.

A piston of suitable length and 0.4-mm diameter is grasped by crocodile forceps and is placed between the incus and the footplate fenestra.

The exact length of the piston is confirmed by performing a hanging and bending test as described by Dr. A. B. R. Desai.

The mobility of the ossicular chain and piston is checked by touching the malleus.

A connective tissue seal is placed around the piston at the fenestra.

The TM flap is reposited back. If the surgery is under local anesthesia, hearing improvement is confirmed by whispering or tuning fork (**Fig. 17.2**).

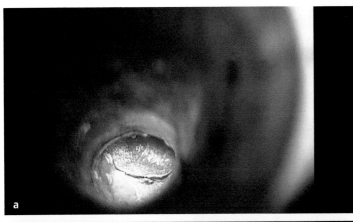

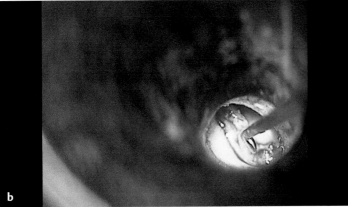

Fig. 17.2 (a) Stapedectomy begins by endomeatal incision. **(b)** Endomeatal incision. Tympanomeatal (TM) flap elevated from the 12 o'clock position to the 6 o'clock position. *(Continued)*

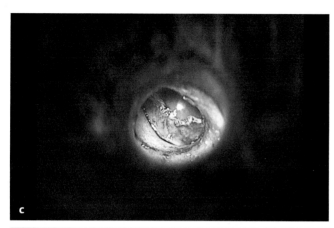

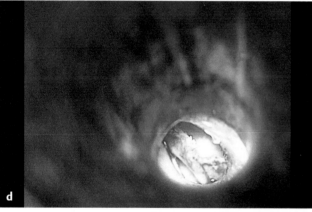

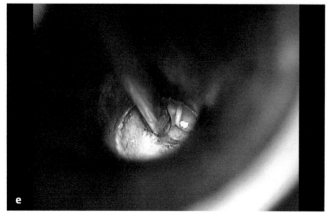

Fig. 17.2 *(Continued)* **(c)** Endomeatal incision. TM flap elevated from the 12 o'clock position to the 6 o'clock position. **(d)** The middle ear is entered just below the level of the chorda tympani nerve. **(e)** Posterosuperior bony meatal wall overhang is removed by 1-mm gauge. *(Continued)*

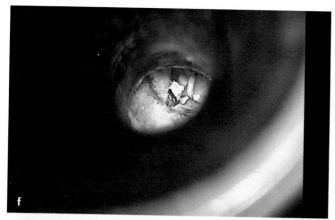

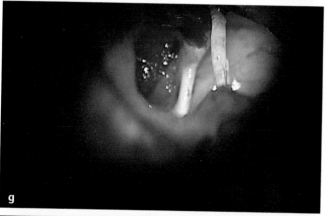

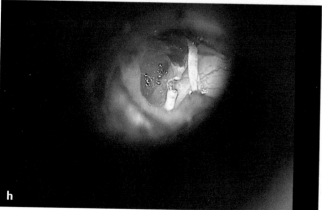

Fig. 17.2 *(Continued)* **(f)** Postero-superior bony meatal wall overhang is removed by 1-mm gauge. **(g)** The stapes area is nicely exposed. The footplate of the stapes is decongested by gelfoam soaked in adrenaline with xylocaine. **(h)** The stapedius muscle is cut by using CO_2 laser beam. *(Continued)*

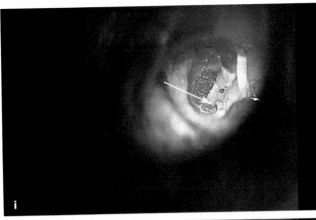

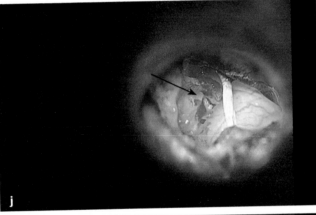

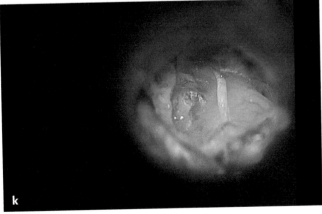

Fig. 17.2 *(Continued)* **(i)** Posterior crura *(arrow)* of the stapes is cut by CO_2 laser beam. **(j, k)** Anterior crura *(arrow)* of the stapes is cut by CO_2 laser beam. *(Continued)*

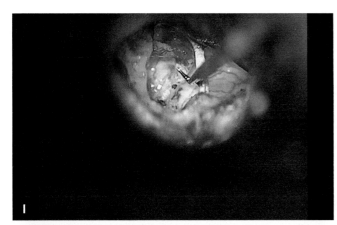

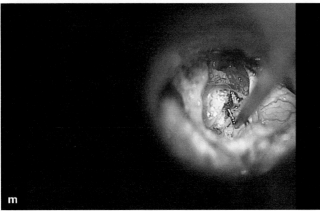

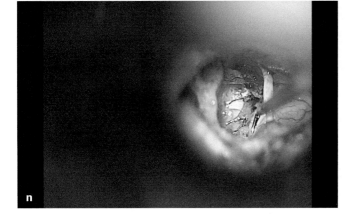

Fig. 17.2 *(Continued)* **(l)** Incudostapedial joint is disarticulated. **(m, n)** The stapes superstructure is removed. *(Continued)*

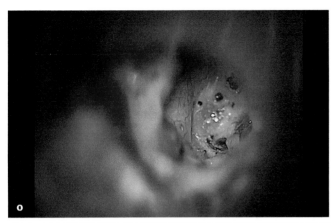

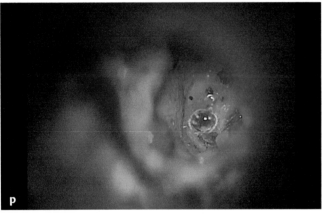

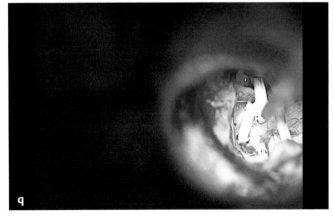

Fig. 17.2 *(Continued)* **(o)** Laser beam is focused over the stapes footplate to make a fenestra. **(p)** A 0.6-mm fenestra is made by CO_2 laser in the posterior part of the stapes footplate. **(q)** A 0.4-mm Teflon piston of proper length is placed and the piston is tightened. *(Continued)*

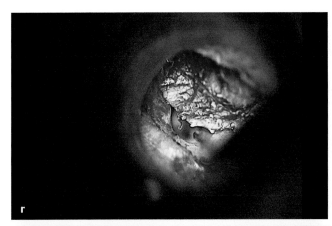

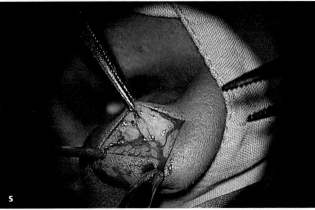

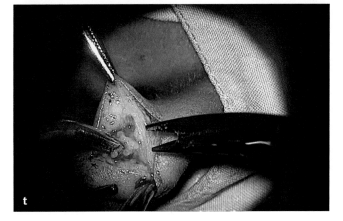

Fig. 17.2 *(Continued)* **(r)** The TM flap is reposited back. In spite of adequate width of the TM flap, it was falling short due to excessive removal of overhang; hence, the TM flap had to be supported by fibrofatty tissue, taken from the lobule of the pinna. **(s, t)** Fibrofatty tissue being removed from the lobule of the pinna. *(Continued)*

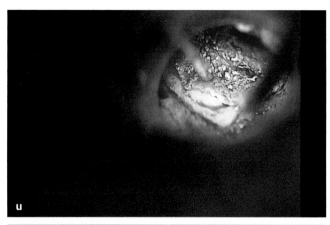

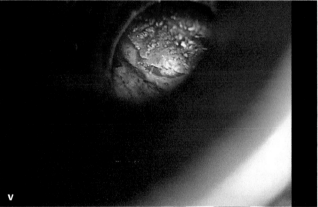

Fig. 17.2 *(Continued)* **(u, v)** The TM flap is being supported by fibrofatty tissue taken out from the lobule of the pinna.

Techniques of Stapes Surgery

There are two techniques in stapes surgery.

- Direct piston technique: Here the stapedotomy of 0.6 mm is made in the posterior part of the footplate and a piston of suitable length and 0.4-mm diameter is placed from the incus (as described earlier; **Fig. 17.3a**).

- Vein graft interposition technique: Here a fenestra of 0.8 mm is made in the posterior part of the footplate. It is covered by a vein graft and a piston of suitable length and 0.4 mm

in diameter is placed between the incus and the indentation in the vein graft at the footplate fenestra. Thus, a large moving surface (0.8 mm) is created with a narrow piston (0.4 mm), which gives maximum range of hearing with maximum closure of the air–bone (AB) gap with no risk of any damage to the utricle and the saccule (**Fig. 17.3b**).

A vein graft of around 0.5 cm is harvested from the dorsum of the hand, its adventitia is thinned out, and the vein is opened.

A small piece of vein graft is to be placed over the footplate fenestra with the intima facing the middle ear.

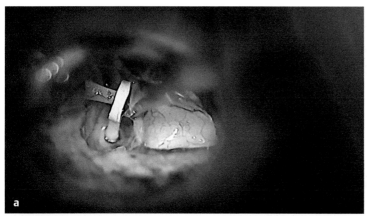

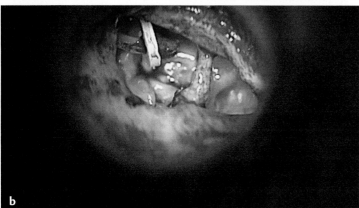

Fig. 17.3 (a) Direct piston technique. (b) Vein graft interposition technique. The fenestra is covered by vein graft and the piston is placed.

The posterior half of the footplate is the most ideal location for making a fenestra.

The distance between the undersurface of the incus and the footplate fenestra is measured, and the length of the piston should be confirmed by a hanging and bending test.

All these measurements are done before placing the vein graft. Then the vein graft is placed over the fenestra and a piston of suitable length and 0.4 mm in diameter is placed between the incus and the indentation in the vein graft at the footplate fenestra. The piston is tightened by crimping it with crocodile forceps.

The mobility of the ossicular chain and the piston is checked by touching the malleus handle.

The TM flap is reposited back and on table hearing is tested. Few pieces of gelfoam are placed in the external auditory canal.

Advantages of the Vein Graft Interposition Technique

- The footplate fenestra is sealed immediately, before placing the piston, which ensures good safety for the inner ear.

- The vein graft is covering the footplate area as well as the promontory, with the intima facing the middle ear. Hence, no raw area is left. Therefore, there is no chance of any adhesions between the lenticular process and the promontory.

- The vein graft prevents the use of overlong piston.

- This technique provides better hearing as the moving surface is 0.8 mm.

Hearing Assessment on OT Table Immediately after Surgery

If the surgery is done under local anesthesia, immediately after repositioning the TM flap, hearing of the patient should always be tested on OT table either by whispering or by performing the tuning fork test.

An audiometry can also be done by headphones, which are covered by a sterilized drape.

If there is no or inadequate improvement in the hearing after repositioning the TM flap, then the following measures are taken:

- Lift up the TM flap again and check for the piston length. If it is found short, it should be changed by proper piston.

- Make the piston tight if it is found to be loose.

- If the piston is found to be touching the edges of the fenestra, then it should be centralized. A discrete fenestra in the posterior part of the footplate with a nice crimping of the piston will help in keeping the piston in the center of the fenestra without touching its edges.

- Check for the mobility of the malleus and the incus. If it was missed earlier, act accordingly.

- Check the round window for its obliteration by an otosclerotic focus, although it is a rare condition.

- Wrong selection of the patient: An audiogram done without proper masking in a patient having unilateral sensorineural hearing loss with a false-negative Rinne in that ear may create such a situation. Hence, a proper Weber test should always be done in these patients before advising surgery. Weber's test done by using a bone conduction vibrator is more reliable.

Hanging Test (as described by Dr. A. B. R. Desai)

This test should be done when the fenestra is of 0.6 mm in diameter and the piston is 0.4 mm thick. A gentle lateral pull is exerted over the incus by a fine right angle hook.

With a gentle lateral pull on the incus, the piston gets hung at the edge of the fenestra. That means the piston is not long (**Fig. 17.4**).

Bending Test

When a gentle lateral pressure is exerted over the piston, it bends. It does not slide over the edge of the fenestra. That means it is not short.

This test is done when the fenestra is of 0.6 mm and the diameter of the piston is 0.4 mm (**Fig. 17.5**).

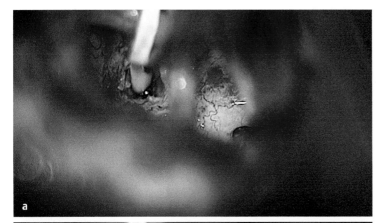

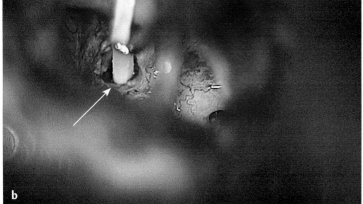

Fig. 17.4 Hanging test. (a) This test is done when the fenestra is of 0.6 mm and the piston is of 0.4 mm. Gentle lateral pull is exerted over the incus by a fine right angle hook. (b) The piston got hung at the edge of the fenestra, which means it is of proper length (*arrow*).

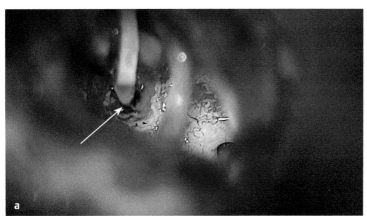

Fig. 17.5 Bending test. (a) It is done when the fenestra is of 0.6 mm and the piston is of 0.4 mm (*arrow*). (*Continued*)

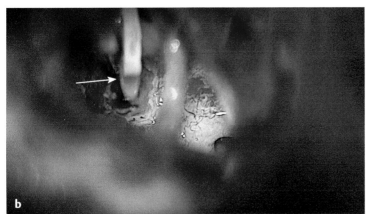

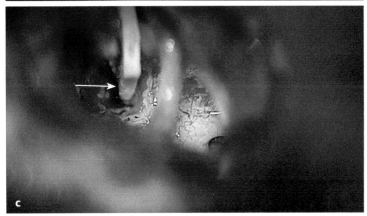

Fig. 17.5 *(Continued)* **(b)** Gentle lateral pressure is exerted over the piston *(arrow)*. **(c)** On gentle lateral pressure, the piston bends *(arrow)*. It does not slide over the edge of the fenestra, which means it is not short.

Stapedectomy with Vein Graft Interposition Technique

Stapedectomy by the vein graft interposition technique is depicted stepwise in **Fig. 17.6**.

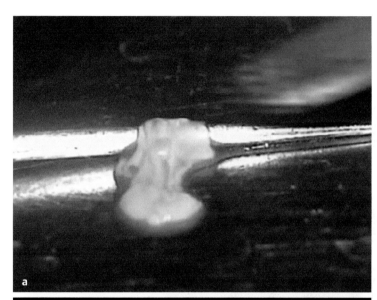

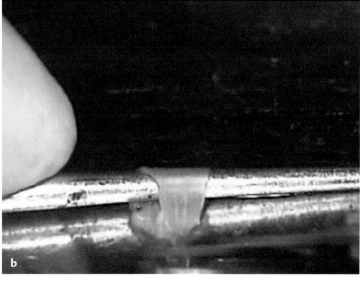

Fig. 17.6 (a) A piece of vein is harvested from the dorsum of the hand. (b) Vein adventitia is thinned out by using a knife. (Continued)

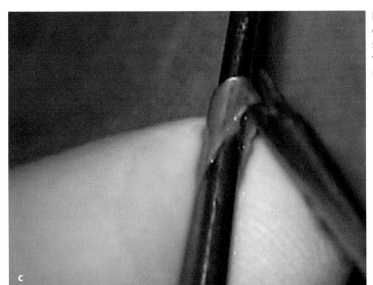

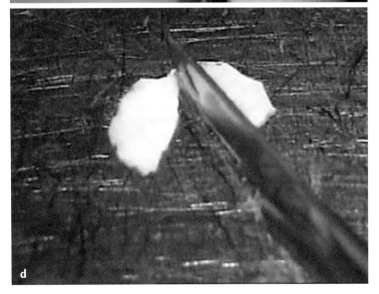

Fig. 17.6 *(Continued)* **(c)** Vein graft is opened by micro-scissors. **(d)** Required size of vein graft piece is selected. *(Continued)*

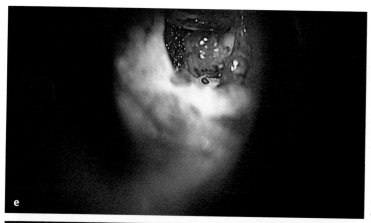

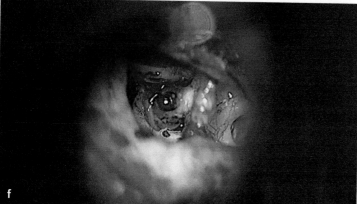

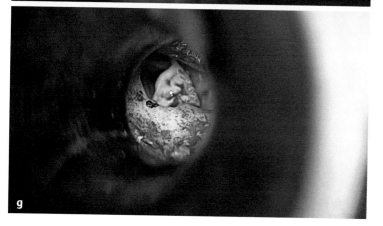

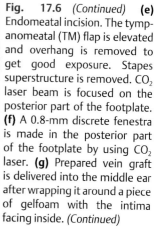

Fig. 17.6 *(Continued)* **(e)** Endomeatal incision. The tympanomeatal (TM) flap is elevated and overhang is removed to get good exposure. Stapes superstructure is removed. CO_2 laser beam is focused on the posterior part of the footplate. **(f)** A 0.8-mm discrete fenestra is made in the posterior part of the footplate by using CO_2 laser. **(g)** Prepared vein graft is delivered into the middle ear after wrapping it around a piece of gelfoam with the intima facing inside. *(Continued)*

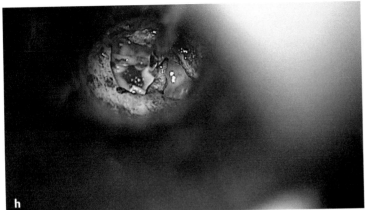

Fig. 17.6 *(Continued)* **(h)** Vein graft, which was wrapped around a piece of gelfoam with the intima facing the middle ear is placed over the footplate fenestra. **(i)** Gelfoam is removed. Vein graft is seen placed over the footplate fenestra with the intima facing the middle ear. **(j)** Footplate fenestra is seen through the thinned-out vein graft. *(Continued)*

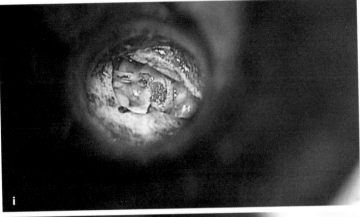

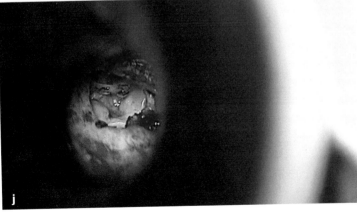

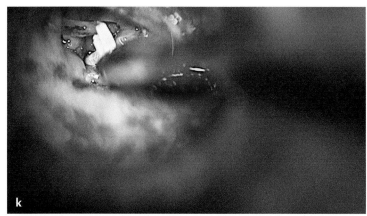

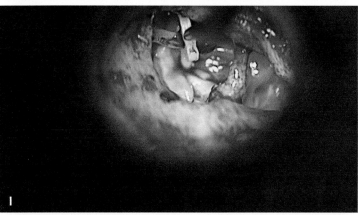

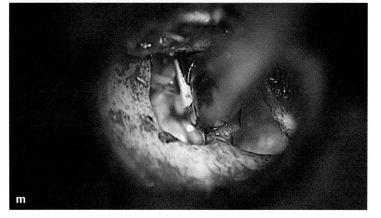

Fig. 17.6 *(Continued)* **(k)** A proper size Teflon piston is placed. **(l)** The piston in position with its lower end into the indentation in the vein graft at the footplate fenestra. **(m)** The piston is tightened by crimping it by using crocodile forceps. *(Continued)*

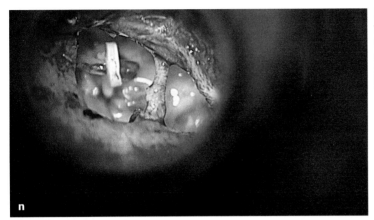

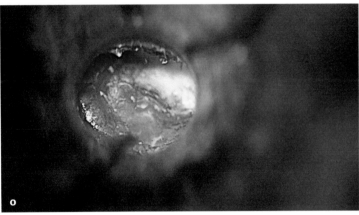

Fig. 17.6 *(Continued)* **(n)** The final position of the vein graft and piston. The piston is exactly at right angle to the footplate. **(o)** The TM flap is reposited back.

Contraindications for Vein Graft Interposition

Vein graft interposition is a very safe technique for stapedectomy giving very stable long-term hearing results, but there are certain contraindications, which are discussed in the following section.

- Vein graft interposition technique is contraindicated in obliterative otosclerosis, as the active otosclerotic focus will grow fast in to mesenchymal tissues of the vein and will cause re-closure of the fenestra.

- In a very deep and narrow oval window niche, the vein graft interposition technique may not be possible.

- It is not possible in cases of dehiscent fallopian canal and ptotic facial nerve, which is lying over the stapes footplate. Footplate exposure can be improved inferiorly by drilling the promontory margins.

- At times, it is difficult to obtain the vein graft especially in obese female patients.

- At times, the patient is not willing for separate incision to be taken for harvesting vein graft.

If the vein graft is not used to cover the footplate fenestra, it means that in direct piston technique, tissues at the fenestra are infiltrated by polymorphs within 24 hours. These polymorphs are then replaced by fibroblasts within 48 hours. The intact membrane of fibrocytes forms within 1 week, and by 3 weeks, firm fibrous membrane is formed. Hence, these 3 weeks are very crucial, and the patient should take all possible precautions during these 3 weeks.

Few Important Tips for the Surgeon

- For effective sound transmission, the piston should be exactly at right angle to the footplate and it should not touch the edges of the fenestra. At times, it is difficult to avoid the piston touching the edges of the fenestra, especially when the piston is not at right angle to the footplate, the possibility of which is very high in a short incus. Here, the piston is a little oblique. Hence, it is better

to make the fenestra a little larger (0.7 mm) to avoid the piston touching its edges even though it is oblique (**Fig. 17.8**).

- The piston should be of proper length. If the piston is longer, no seal of any kind will prevent the perilymph fistula, as the leak is always submucosal. The length of the piston required is to be customized as per the patient. One size cannot be used for all the patients. The range of piston required for various patients is 3.25 to 4.75 mm. The length of the piston should be perfect, as the utricle and the saccule is 0.8 to 1 mm from the footplate and any inward displacement of the prosthesis due to positive pressure in the external auditory canal or due to barotrauma will perforate the saccule or the utricle.

Fig. 17.8 (a) Piston touching the edges of the fenestra (*arrow*). **(b)** The piston is centralized. It is not touching the edges of the fenestra. It is at right angle to the footplate.

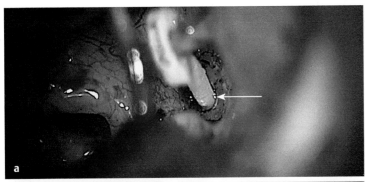

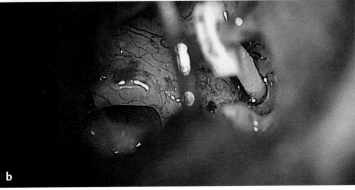

- Regarding the location of fenestra, earlier the posterior third of the footplate was considered the safest area for making a fenestra, but now it is confirmed that the middle third of footplate, especially its inferior part, is the safest area as the distance between the footplate and the membranous labyrinth is maximum (0.8–1.00 mm) here.

- Firm crimping of the piston is essential to get perfect closure of the AB gap. Do not rely on the memory effect of the Teflon piston. Firm crimping of the piston does not lead to incus necrosis. It is the tight crimping that is not desirable. Proper discrete fenestra and firm crimping are essential to prevent migration of the prosthesis.

- At any cost, the surgeon should never take his suction tip near the footplate fenestra. Accidental suction of the perilymph should be avoided.

- In the direct piston technique, few drops of blood at the fenestra as a seal are also used. The blood gets clotted within a few minutes and this clotted blood is made up of fibrin, which acts as a stronger tissue seal. Blood clot forms an effective seal under and around the piston (**Fig. 17.9**).

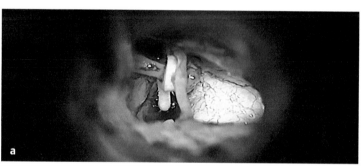

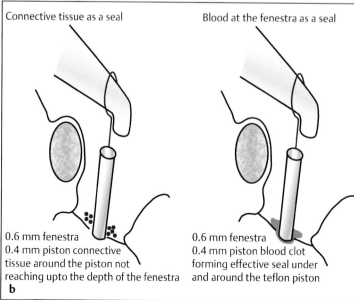

Fig. 17.9 (a, b) Blood is used as effective seal around the piston at the fenestra.

Connective tissue as a seal   Blood at the fenestra as a seal

0.6 mm fenestra
0.4 mm piston connective tissue around the piston not reaching upto the depth of the fenestra

0.6 mm fenestra
0.4 mm piston blood clot forming effective seal under and around the teflon piston

18 Reverse Stapedotomy

The reverse stapedotomy consists of making the stapes footplate fenestra first, with the introduction of a piston and crimping of the piston before removal of the stapes superstructure.

This reverse stapedotomy helps in making the fenestra in the stapes footplate without any risk of subluxation of the stapes footplate or without any risk of a floating footplate as the stapes is well supported by the intact incudostapedial (IS) joint.

This also prevents incus subluxation or excessive movement of the piston into the vestibule while crimping the piston because the incus is stabilized by intact IS joint.

The reverse stapedotomy may not be possible in all the cases as there may not be any working space between the fallopian canal and the stapes superstructure in many patients and the stapes footplate is hidden.

It is not possible in cases of dehiscent fallopian canal and ptotic facial nerve. Here there is no space to make the fenestra in the stapes footplate, before removal of the stapes superstructure (**Fig. 18.1**).

Fig. 18.2 depicts the steps involved in reverse stapedotomy.

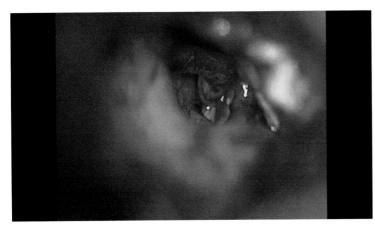

Fig. 18.1 No working space between the fallopian canal and the stapes superstructure. The stapes footplate is hidden.

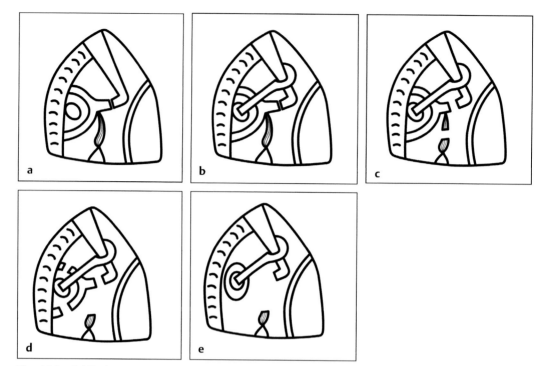

Fig. 18.2 **(a)** Exploratory tympanotomy of the right ear. The mobility of all the ossicles were tested, Here the stapes is fixed. A 0.6-mm fenestra is made in the stapes footplate, before cutting the stapedius tendon, before separating the incudostapedial joint and before removing the stapes superstructure. **(b)** A Teflon piston of proper length and diameter (0.4 mm) is placed between the incus and the footplate fenestra, and is tightened by crimping. **(c)** The stapedius muscle is cut and the incudostapedial joint is separated. **(d)** The stapes superstructure is fractured and removed. **(e)** The mobility of the ossicles and the piston is checked, and the tympanomeatal flap is reposited.

19 Postoperative Treatment

Postoperative Treatment Protocols

Postoperative treatment includes careful adherence to the following protocols:

- Patient should rest in a propped-up position for a day. He should avoid lying on the operated ear for a few days. He should not make any sudden and violent head movements as it will precipitate vertigo.

- Antibiotics and analgesics should be given; if necessary, labyrinthine sedatives are to be given.

- The patient should be discharged next day if there is no vertigo.

- After discharge the patient should be advised the following:

  o Not to blow his nose.

  o Avoid straining (not to lift heavy weights).

  o Not to do any violent head movements as it causes dizziness.

  o Immediate treatment of cold if he gets it.

Postoperative Vertigo

Vertigo following stapedectomy is not uncommon. Minor vertigo remains for a day or two, due to labyrinthine reaction to surgical trauma, which resolves very soon. Similarly entry of blood and air in the vestibule resolves within 2 to 3 days. These patients should be given labyrinthine sedatives for few days. Severe vertigo remaining for a longer period of time associated with decreased hearing could be due to inner ear trauma due to rough handling of the footplate by an inexperience surgeon. These patients should be given steroid for a week or 10 days along with labyrithine sedatives. Usually these patients settle down but some degree of sensorineural hearing loss remains depending upon the severity of labyrinthine insult.

For persistent vertigo with decreased or fluctuating hearing loss with tinnitus, there is the possibility of a perilymph fistula and it should be managed accordingly.

Postoperative Facial Nerve Palsy

Facial nerve palsy during stapedectomy is not common. At times, temporary immediate facial nerve palsy occurs due to local anesthesia, which at times block the nerve at the stylomastoid foramen. This palsy usually recovers within 3 to 4 hours.

If the palsy persists for more than 3 to 4 hours after surgery, then the possibility of nerve getting damaged during surgery is very high. Generation of heat at the footplate of the stapes due to drilling or due to laser causes edema of the facial nerve with palsy, which takes few weeks to recover. This patient should be given high dose of steroids for 10 days. If the surgeon is very much sure that he has not damaged the nerve, these cases should be managed conservatively. If surgeon is not sure about the nerve integrity, it should be explored.

Major injury to the facial nerve is rare in stapedectomy, but can occur in revision cases where the footplate area is covered by fibrous tissue, and any manipulation in this area can damage the facial nerve especially when the nerve is dehiscent and bulging down over the stapes footplate area.

20 Microdrill for Stapedotomy: An Essential Tool

Introduction

Among all the steps, two steps in the stapedectomy are very important.

- Making a proper fenestra in the footplate: Making a fenestra in the footplate of the stapes by pick exerts pressure over the footplate and may cause either subluxation of the footplate or a floating footplate especially when it is not fixed adequately (**Fig. 20.1**).

- Removal of the stapes superstructure: Fracturing the crura of the stapes by the pressure of the right-angle hook is a very crude procedure and can cause removal of the stapes in toto, which is very dangerous and can lead to a dead ear (**Fig. 20.2**).

These accidents make the surgery eventful and the patient can lose hearing.

Chances of getting all these complications are very high under the following circumstances:

- When the footplate of the stapes is not properly fixed (early otosclerosis).

- When the footplate is diffusely thickened, but the margins (annular ligament) are weak (biscuit footplate).

To avoid all these complications, the microdrill plays a very important role. The microdrill is nothing but a small size stapedotomy micro-drill system having a powerful high-tech micro-motor that rotates at a speed of 2,000 to 6,000 rpm, with absolutely no vibrations and no jerks. It is an essential tool for stapedotomy.

The microdrill handpiece is small in size, very light (60 g), and easy to handle. The front tip is long curved, allowing easy access to the stapes footplates. The long slender front portion allows you to work

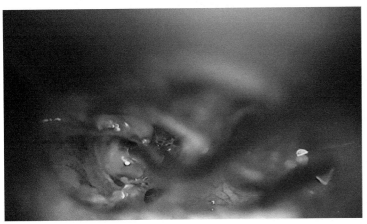

Fig. 20.1 Floating footplate.

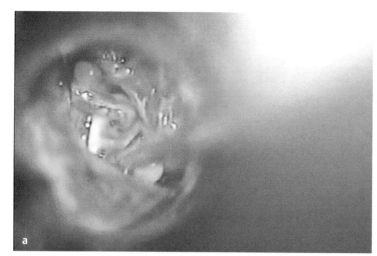

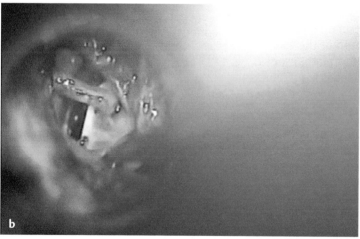

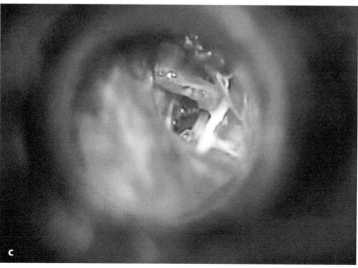

Fig. 20.2 **(a)** Removal of the stapes in toto caused by the pressure of the right angle hook. **(b)** Removal of the stapes in toto. **(c)** Complete removal of the stapes; oval window is fully exposed.

through the ear speculum, so that surgery can be done through an endomeatal incision comfortably. A penlike grip gives easier and better skill for crucial working at the stapes footplate (**Fig. 20.3**).

It is easily washable and can withstand repeated autoclaving.

The microdrill is very much essential for cases of obliterative otosclerosis to make the fenestra.

A routine micro-motor with angled handpiece with diamond bur (0.6 mm) can also be used in place of the microdrill, but it is full of vibrations and is not an ideal instrument for stapedotomy (**Fig. 20.4**).

Other uses of the microdrills are the following:

- For removal of bony overhang (posterosuperior bony canal wall) by using a cutting bur.

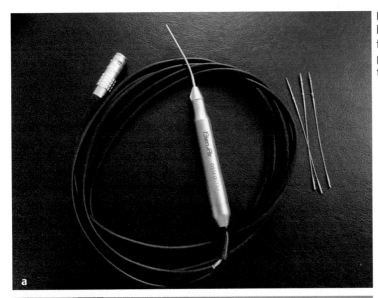

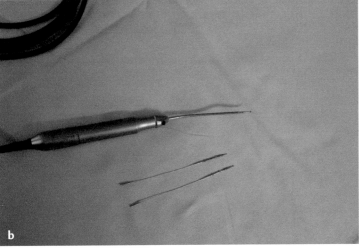

Fig. 20.3 (a) Microdrill with burs. **(b)** Microdrill with the bur fitted. The long slender front portion allows you to work through the ear speculum.

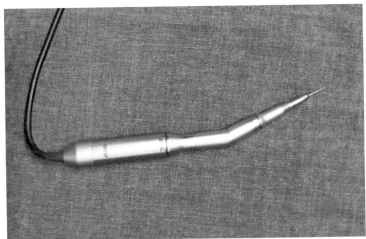

Fig. 20.4 A micro-motor with an angled handpiece with a diamond bur.

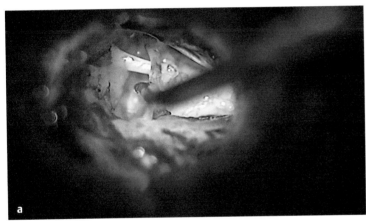

Fig. 20.5 (a) The middle ear is opened by an endomeatal incision. The posterosuperior overhang is removed. The mucosa over the footplate of the stapes is removed, exposing it, for drilling by microdrill. *(Continued)*

- It can also be used for the removal of the malleus head by drilling the neck of the malleus, in cases of tympanoplasty when the malleus head nipper is not available.

Microdrill Stapedotomy

Steps of the microdrill stapedotomy are showcased in **Fig. 20.5**.

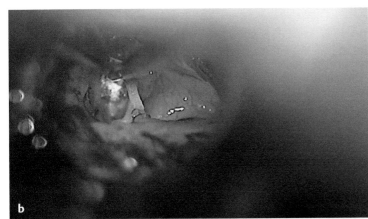

Fig. 20.5 *(Continued)* **(b)** The mucosa over the stapes footplate is effectively removed by gently rubbing the footplate by gelfoam. **(c)** The footplate of the stapes is demucosalized. Raw footplate is seen. **(d)** Microdrill with a diamond bur of 0.6 mm is used to drill the footplate as well as the posterior crura. *(Continued)*

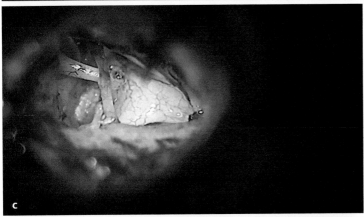

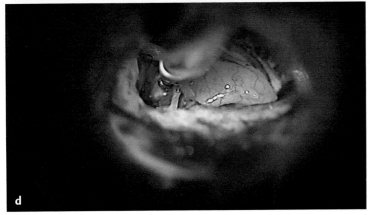

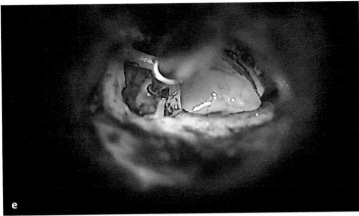

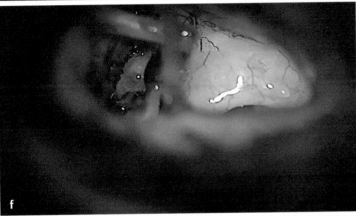

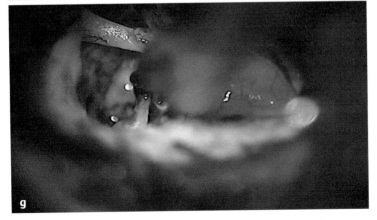

Fig. 20.5 *(Continued)* **(e)** The footplate is *blue-lined*. The posterior crura is completely drilled. **(f)** The footplate of the stapes is *blue-lined*. **(g)** The stapedius muscle is divided by scissors. *(Continued)*

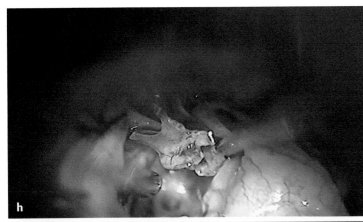

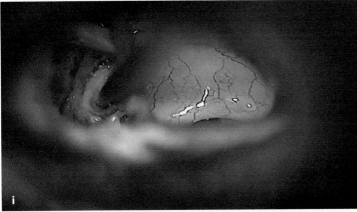

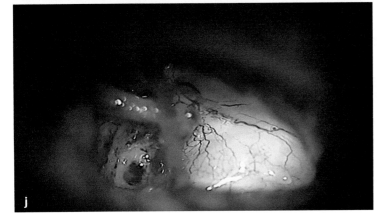

Fig. 20.5 *(Continued)* **(h)** The incudostapedial (IS) joint separated. The stapes superstructure is removed by fracturing the anterior crura. **(i)** The fenestra is made in the footplate by a straight pick. **(j)** The footplate fenestra is made by a straight pick. Small bony pieces are removed. *(Continued)*

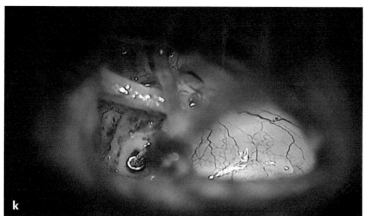

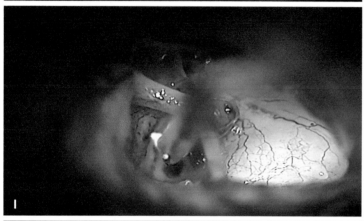

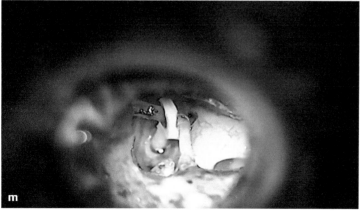

Fig. 20.5 *(Continued)* **(k)** The fenestra in the stapes footplate is enlarged to 0.6 mm. **(l)** Distance between the stapes footplate and the incus is measured. **(m)** A proper size piston is placed. *(Continued)*

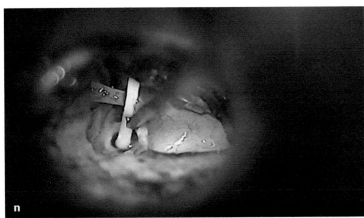

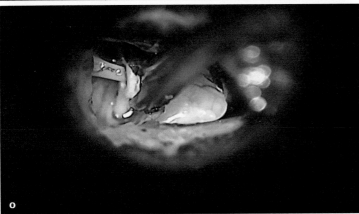

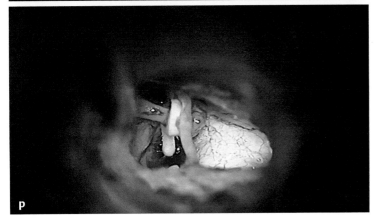

Fig. 20.5 *(Continued)* **(n)** The hanging test is done to confirm the length of the piston. **(o)** The piston is tightened by crimping it by crocodile forceps. **(p)** Few drops of blood is used as tissue seal. *(Continued)*

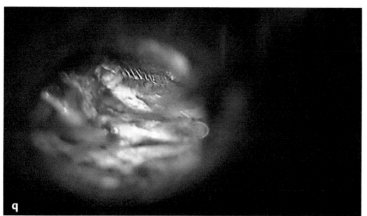

Fig. 20.5 *(Continued)* **(q)** The tympanomeatal flap is reposited back.

Conclusion

The microdrill is an ideal instrument for stapedotomy. It is a very safe tool for making fenestra in the stapes footplate and for the removal of the stapes superstructure. As per the author, every stapes surgeon should have it on his instrument trolley.

21 Large Fenestra versus Small Fenestra

Introduction

It is mentioned earlier that the procedure in the past was stapedectomy (large fenestra surgery) in which near-total removal of the stapes footplate was done. Nowadays, the procedure done is stapedotomy (small fenestra surgery). Stapedotomy is an innovation over stapedectomy.

In stapedotomy, a small fenestra of 0.6 mm is made in the posterior part of the footplate with a 0.4-mm-thick piston is used. This is a very safe as the utricle and saccule are situated around 0.8 mm away from this part of the footplate and there is no chance of any trauma to these structures. Recent findings suggest that the middle third of footplate, especially its inferior part, is very safe for stapedotomy.

Large Fenestra Surgery: Stapedectomy

In stapedectomy, there is a good immediate improvement in the hearing following surgery and good closure of the air–bone (AB) gap, but surgery here is very much traumatic to the inner ear. Postoperative, the patient is very much symptomatic and it takes more time for his vertigo to settle down.

There are more number of cases of late decline in the hearing due to sensorineural deafness, which could be due to trauma to the inner ear or perilymph fistula formation, which is very common with bigger fenestrae.

Small Fenestra Surgery: Stapedotomy

Stapedotomy is very safe as it is less traumatic to the inner ear and has fewer complications.

Both immediate and late hearing results are very stable with small fenestra surgeries. Now with the availability of microdrill and laser, small fenestra surgery (stapedotomy) is a very regular procedure (**Fig. 21.1**).

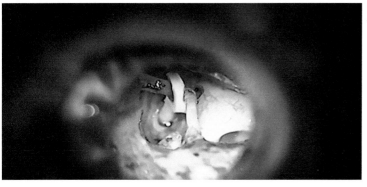

Fig. 21.1 Stapedotomy (small fenestra surgery).

22 Reconstruction of the Stapedius Muscle

Introduction

Routinely during stapedectomy, the stapedius muscle is cut and is not reconstructed. These patients remain unhappy for few months, even though there is a good closure of the air–bone gap and there is good improvement in the hearing. The cause for this unhappiness is intolerance to the loud sounds like the sounds of horn, utensils, child crying, etc.

Hence, the stapedius muscle should be reconstructed after stapedectomy. This restores the normal physiological protective effect of muscle on the prosthesis.

In the normal ear, on exposure to loud sounds, the stapedius muscle contracts. It rotates the footplate around its transverse axis and thus stretches the annular ligament. The stapedius and tensor tympani muscle contraction decreases the transmission of sound waves, by increasing the stiffness of the ossicular chain.

Surgical Steps

The stapedius muscle is not cut; it is detached from the stapes by a sharp sickle knife so that you get a full length of the stapedius muscle.

After completing the stapedotomy, after placing the piston, a small piece of connective tissue or vein graft is placed between cut end of the stapedius muscle and the incus. Gradually, it gets vascularized and becomes a full muscle, attached to the incus.

Contraction of this muscle increases the stiffness of the ossicular chain (not proved).

The advantages of a stapedius muscle reconstruction are the following:

- The blood supply of the lenticular process of the incus via the stapedius muscle is maintained.

- It also supports the prosthesis preventing its migration.

- On exposure to loud sounds, the stapedius muscle contracts, which increases the stiffness of the middle ear ossicles and thus reduces hyperacusis. Such a patient can tolerate noise better.

- Tympanometry in these patients shows an increase in impedance. A change in the impedance of tympanic membrane has been observed, but the impedance change at the oval window membrane could not be studied.

- Causse, in 1997, claimed to show improved speech intelligibility in noise and reduced intolerance of loud noise after reconstructing the stapedius muscle during stapedectomy.

Conclusion

The results of various studies show that these patients are very happy. They do not have any discomfort when they are exposed to loud sounds; hence, the author feels that everybody should follow this small procedure.

Fig. 22.1 shows the reconstruction of the stapedius muscle during stapedectomy.

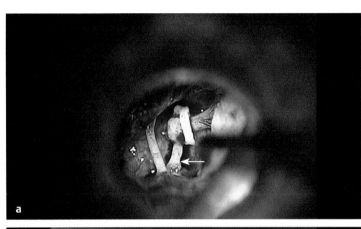

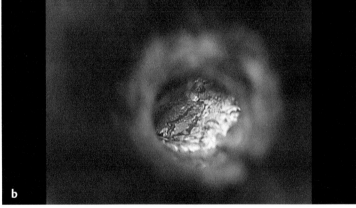

Fig. 22.1 **(a)** While performing a stapedectomy, the stapedius muscle is preserved, and connective tissue is placed between the stapedius muscle and the incus after placing a Teflon piston. One end of the connective tissue overlaps the stapedius muscle and the other end is placed around the incus. The *arrow* shows the stapedius muscle with connective tissue overlapping it. **(b)** The tympanomeatal flap is reposited back.

23 Loose Piston Over the Incus

Introduction

Firm attachment of the prosthesis to the long process of the incus is necessary for effective sound transmission. Many a time, the incus is thin, and the loop of the piston is bigger; hence, some gap remains between the piston and the incus, in spite of crimping of the piston nicely. This makes effective sound transmission impossible. Even when a very good stapedectomy is done, some air–bone gap remains. These patients are unhappy, as some deafness is still persisting.

To overcome this limitation, it is advisable to use a Teflon piston with a narrow loop, or Shea's piston having a loop with an inner diameter of 0.63 mm (**Fig. 23.1**).

Use of a Teflon wire prosthesis or titanium prosthesis is also encouraged so that one can tighten the piston as per need (**Fig. 23.2**). But this one is costly.

A simple method that the author uses to tighten the piston is to use the chorda tympani nerve. The chorda tympani nerve is completely mobilized and gently slided into the loop of the Teflon piston. Thus, the gap between the loop of the Teflon piston and the incus is filled up by the nerve so that the piston comes in close contact with the incus, without disturbing the nerve function of the chorda tympani (**Fig. 23.3**).

Results

Hearing results in these patients are compared by doing an intraoperative audiometry by using headphones covered by sterilized drapes. The air–bone gap of 20 to 25 dB that was there before, due to a loose piston, disappeared after putting the chorda into the loop of the Teflon piston, that is, after making the piston tight (**Fig. 23.4**).

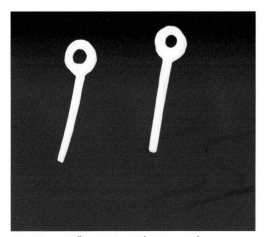

Fig. 23.1 Teflon piston with a narrow loop.

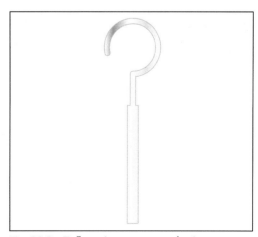

Fig. 23.2 Teflon wire stapes prosthesis.

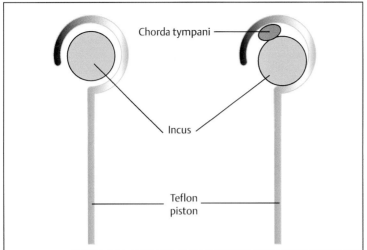

Fig. 23.3 Chorda tympani nerve slided under the loop of a teflon piston.

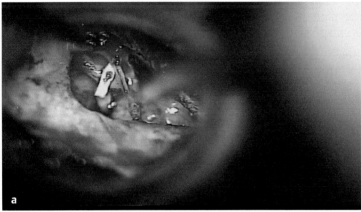

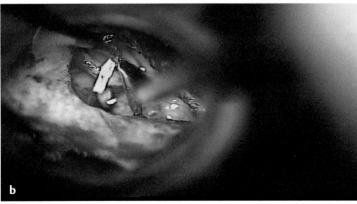

Fig. 23.4 (a) Stapedotomy is completed, the piston is placed, and the chorda tympani nerve is mobilized completely. **(b)** The chorda tympani nerve is slided into the loop of the Teflon piston, which is loose in spite of a tight crimping. *(Continued)*

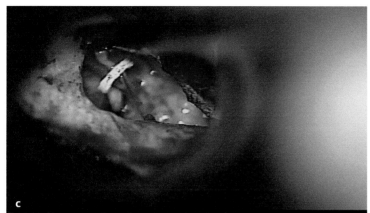

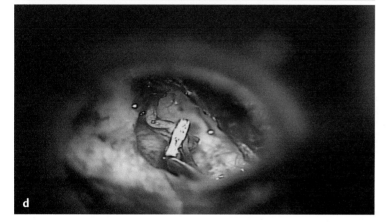

Fig. 23.4 *(Continued)* **(c, d)** The gap between the loop of the Teflon piston and the incus is filled up by the nerve so that the piston comes in close contact with the incus, leading to improvement in hearing.

24 Problems during Stapedectomy

Introduction

Usually, there are no problems during stapedectomy. Certain anatomical and physiological variations are encountered, which makes surgery difficult, and the surgeon should be prepared to handle these difficult situations. Various problems during stapedectomy are the following:

- Narrow external auditory canal and bulging bony canal wall (big overhang).
- Thin, delicate meatal wall skin.
- Dehiscent facial nerve and facial nerve injury.
- Bleeding during surgery.
- Floating footplate.
- Perilymph flooding.
- Persistent stapedial artery.
- Obliterative otosclerosis.
- Malleus head fixation.
- Incus necrosis/absent incus/short incus with otosclerosis.
- Deep and narrow oval window niche.

Narrow External Auditory Canal and Bulging Canal Wall (Big Overhang)

This is a very common situation, making it difficult to expose the stapes area. In this situation, if it is found difficult to perform the surgery by endomeatal incision, it is better to start the surgery with endaural incision rather than struggling with endomeatal incision.

The endaural incision required here is relatively small than the classical bigger endaural incision.

A big posterosuperior canal wall overhang requires removal by a good curette or a micro-drill with diamond bur. A small gauge (1 mm) with a hammer is also an effective way of removing the canal wall overhang gently (**Fig. 24.1**).

Thin, Delicate Meatal Wall Skin

At times, the meatal skin is very thin and delicate without much periosteal support. It is difficult to elevate such skin intact and equally difficult to reposit it as there are high chances of tearing of skin. Here the surgeon has to be very slow and gentle.

Dehiscence of the Fallopian Canal (0.5%) and Facial Nerve Injury

After opening the middle ear and while palpating the ossicular chain, attention should always be given to the fallopian canal, which may be dehiscent. At times, this dehiscent facial nerve bulges down over the stapes crura, thus hiding the stapes footplate (**Fig. 24.2**).

If the bulge is less and not hiding the footplate of the stapes, surgery can be performed in a normal way with due care and no instrument should touch the facial nerve accidently. At times, the nerve is partially exposed, especially the inferior surface.

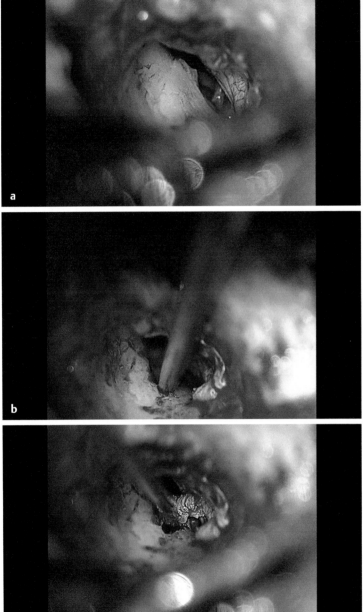

Fig. 24.1 **(a)** Big postero-superior canal wall overhang hiding the stapes and the incus. **(b)** Very effective way of removal of the posterosuperior overhang is by using a 1-mm gauge and hammer. **(c)** Bony pieces removed. *(Continued)*

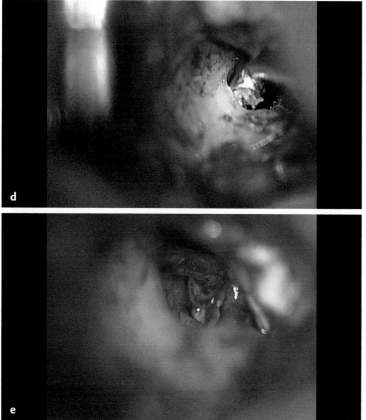

Fig. 24.1 *(Continued)* **(d)** Big overhang removal by a curette, which is required for adequate exposure of the stapes area. **(e)** Big posterosuperior overhang being removed for good exposure to the stapes area.

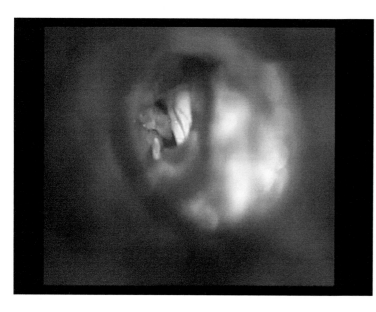

Fig. 24.2 Dehiscent facial nerve touching the stapes crura. The stapes footplate is not seen.

If the bulge is hiding the stapes footplate, little extension is given to the neck of the patient to expose the footplate area and complete the procedure.

If the bulge is moderate, the procedure can be completed by drilling the footplate close to the promontory and making a fenestra at the inferior margin of the footplate. This can only be performed by an experienced surgeon. In both situations, a bucket handle prosthesis is ideal, as it fits to the tip of the lenticular process of the incus far below the dehiscent facial nerve.

If the bulge is severe and the procedure is going to be risky, abandon the procedure. It is advisable to give hearing aid to this patient.

Chorda Tympani Nerve during Stapedectomy

Regarding the chorda tympani nerve, attempts are always made to preserve the nerve during a stapes surgery. If the nerve is stretched too much, it is better to transect it, as there is no long-term loss of taste sensation if the nerve is transected. A transected nerve causes short-term symptoms that improve within 3 to 6 months. A stretched nerve is more disturbing as it causes long-term unpleasant metallic taste and impairment of taste sensation, which is very disturbing. Symptoms are more when the nerve is damaged in both the ears.

Bleeding during Surgery

Surgery done under local anesthesia, by using 1 or 2% xylocaine with 1:100,000 adrenaline is very effective in making the surgery bloodless by providing good vasoconstriction.

Once the footplate is exposed, it is very important to decongest the mucosa of the stapes footplate by using gelfoam soaked in xylocaine with adrenaline. Put the gelfoam there for 7 minutes. Maintain the pressure by putting small dry gelfoam over the wet Gelfoam. Once the footplate mucosa is decongested nicely, demucosalize the footplate to prevent any bleeding.

If the decongestion is not done properly, especially in the cases where the mucosa is very much hypertrophied and vascular, troublesome bleeding is likely to be there the moment the mucosa is touched. If the bleeding occurs after a fenestra is made in the footplate, it is going to complicate the situation.

If bleeding occurs before making the fenestra, it is controlled by repacking the footplate by gelfoam soaked in 1:20,000 adrenaline and allowed to wait for some time. If blood pressure is found to be on the higher side during surgery, it should be controlled by intravenous (IV) nitroglycerine (NTG) in titrating doses. This will safely maintain the blood pressure on the lower side so that the surgeon gets a clean, dry field and can perform the surgery peacefully.

Now CO_2 laser, in coagulation mode, is used to coagulate all the bleeding points in the mucosa over and around the stapes footplate. Even the bony bleeding from the otosclerosis focus can also be coagulated by CO_2 laser during surgery (**Fig. 24.3**).

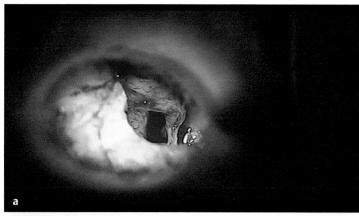

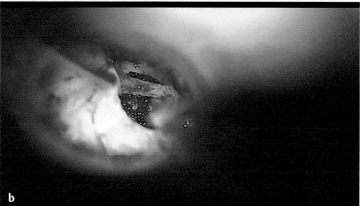

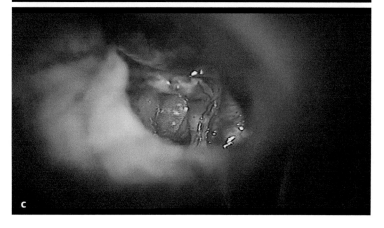

Fig. 24.3 **(a)** Markedly hypertrophied footplate mucosa, which bleeds on touch. **(b)** Bleeding temporarily stops by the pressure of gelfoam. **(c)** For effectively stopping the bleeding from the footplate mucosa, CO_2 laser in coagulation mode is very useful. *(Continued)*

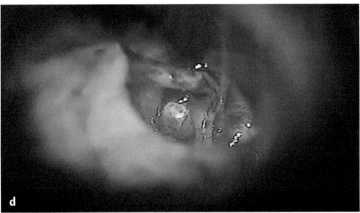

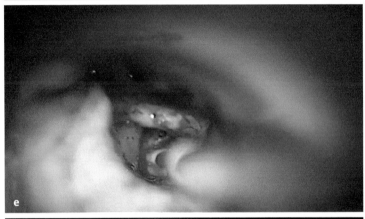

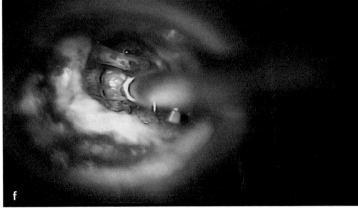

Fig.   24.3 *(Continued)* **(d)** Bleeding vessels in the footplate mucosa are coagulated by CO_2 laser. **(e)** The footplate is exposed after removing the decongested mucosa. The footplate is drilled by the microdrill. The microdrill is used to saucerize and *blue line* the footplate. **(f)** The footplate is nicely saucerized and *blue lined*. *(Continued)*

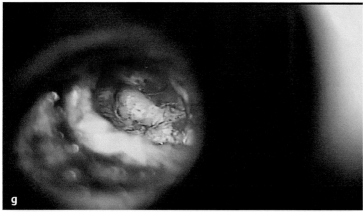

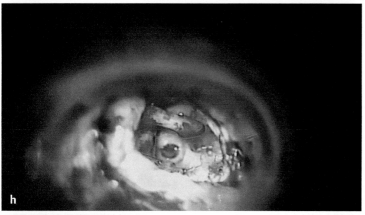

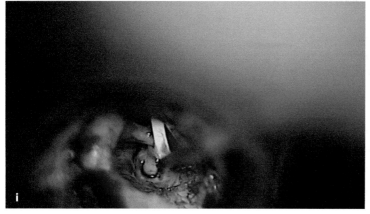

Fig. 24.3 *(Continued)* **(g)** Laser beam is focused over the posterior half of the footplate. **(h)** A 0.6-mm fenestra is made in the posterior part of the footplate by CO_2 laser. **(i)** A 0.4-mm piston is placed exactly at right angle to the footplate. *(Continued)*

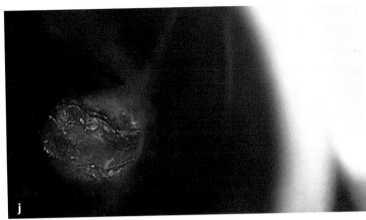

Fig. 24.3 *(Continued)* **(j)** A tympanomeatal flap is reposited back after crimping the piston.

Fig. 24.4 depicts another case where the footplate mucosa was again highly vascular and was bleeding on touch. These bleeding vessels are coagulated by coagulation mode of CO_2 laser. Footplate fenestra is made by CO_2 laser.

Incus Subluxation

Enough care should always be taken to prevent this subluxation of incus during stapedectomy. Subluxation of the incus can occur during the following steps:

- While removing the posterosuperior bony canal wall overhang, due to accidental slipping of the curette or gauge.

- While separating the incudostapedial joint.

- During firm crimping of the piston over the incus.

If subluxation is minor and all the attachments of the incus are not broken, the procedure can be completed, but it is difficult and challenging to put the prosthesis on the subluxated incus, as the incus is not stable and may get dislocated while putting the piston. Hence, due care should be taken while placing the prosthesis (piston) over the subluxated incus.

If there is a major subluxation or complete dislocation of the incus, it can be reposited back into its original position, well supported by gelfoam. The tympanomeatal flap is reposited and ear is reexplored after 6 months.

The other alternative is to remove the subluxated or dislocated incus, remove the head of the malleus by cutting it at the neck by the malleus head nipper, and perform malleostapedotomy, which can be done during same sitting only.

The Floating Footplate

There is sudden dislodgement of the stapes footplate from the surrounding oval window niche, even when the slightest of pressure is exerted on it.

Chances of getting this complication are very high in the following conditions:

- In early otosclerosis, when the footplate is minimally fixed and get dislodged or become mobile with the minimum pressure of pick or perforator.

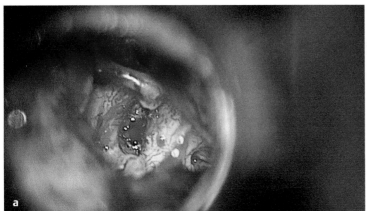

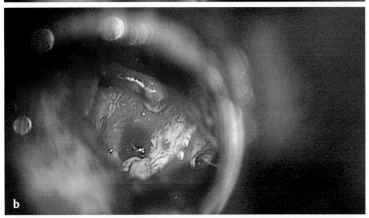

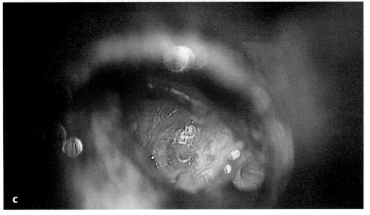

Fig. 24.4 (a, b) Bleeding vessels on the stapes footplate. **(c)** Bleeding vessels on the stapes footplate are coagulated by the coagulation mode of CO_2 laser. *(Continued)*

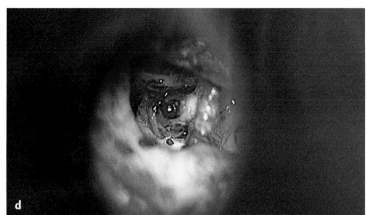

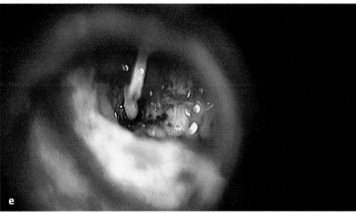

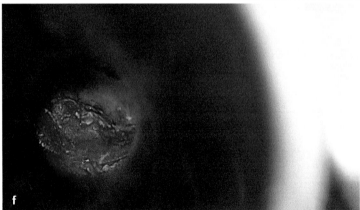

Fig. 24.4 *(Continued)* **(d)** A 0.6-mm fenestra is made in the posterior part of the footplate, by a single shot of CO_2 laser. **(e)** A proper size piston is placed and tightened. **(f)** The tympanomeatal flap is reposited back.

- When the stapes footplate is diffusely thickened, but the annular ligament is weak (biscuit footplate) and get dislodged with the slightest of pressure exerted over the footplate by pick, perforator, or even microdrill.

The best thing to do to prevent the occurrence of this complication is by making the footplate fenestra before removal of the stapes superstructure (reverse stapedotomy).

If the floating footplate occurs after removal of the stapes superstructure and it is difficult to remove the footplate atraumatically, no further attempt should be made to remove the footplate. The best thing is to put a Teflon piston between the incus and the floating footplate and put connective tissue around the piston. A perfect length of teflon piston is required for good contact between the piston and the footplate (**Fig. 24.5**).

If the footplate enters deep into the vestibule, nothing can be done. The best thing is to plug the oval window with connective tissue and abandon the procedure. This patient may end up with severe vertigo with sensorineural hearing loss (SNHL).

If there is facility of CO_2 laser, the best thing is to make the fenestra in the floating stapes footplate by laser (atraumatic) and put a proper size piston between the incus and the fenestra.

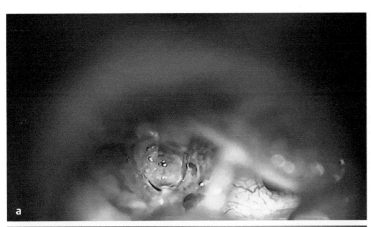

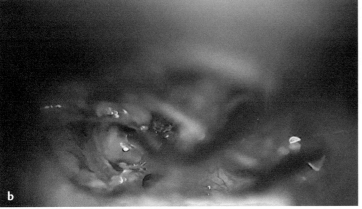

Fig. 24.5 (a) A floating footplate. **(b)** The distance between the incus and the floating footplate is measured. *(Continued)*

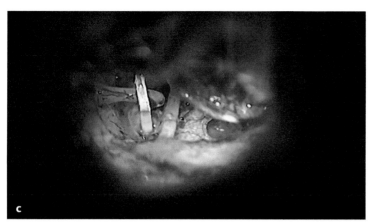

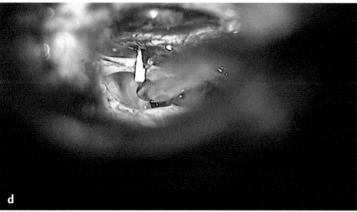

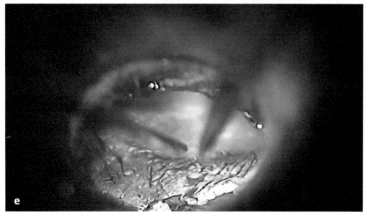

Fig. 24.5 *(Continued)* **(c)** A proper size piston is placed between the incus and the floating footplate. **(d)** The piston is tightened by crimping it by crocodile forceps. **(e)** The tympanomeatal flap is reposited back after putting the connective tissue around the piston.

If floating footplate occurs before removal of the stapes superstructure (during reverse stapedotomy), nothing should be done. It is better to close and come out.

A floating footplate is least likely to occur when the laser is used to create the fenestra.

Depressed Footplate in the Vestibule

At times while making the fenestra, the footplate (complete or part of it) may get depressed into the vestibule, especially if the pick or perforator used during surgery is blunt. It is better to abandon the procedure at that moment rather than making any attempt for extraction of the footplate and further exploration is to be done at a higher center where there is CO_2 laser facility (**Fig. 24.6**).

Perilymph Flooding or Gusher (1:500)

Perilymph gushes out when the vestibule is open. These gushers may be minor or major (profuse).

Minor gushers (oozers) are due to abnormally patent cochlear aqueduct causing cerebrospinal fluid (CSF) to flow through the cochlea into the vestibule.

Major gushers are due to some dehiscence at the fundus of internal auditory canal.

Both these conditions can be demonstrated preoperatively by a computed tomography (CT) scan of the temporal bone done in both axial and coronal planes, which will most likely show an abnormally patent cochlear aqueduct and dysplasia of internal auditory canal and the cochlea.

The perilymph gusher is very common in cases of congenital fixation of the stapes.

Treatment

If it occurs, there is no need to get panicked. Wait for some time, perilymph flooding becomes less and the procedure can be completed especially in minor gushers. Otherwise following steps should be taken:

- Raising the head end of the operation table to reduce CSF pressure.

- IV mannitol is given to reduce CSF pressure. If perilymph pressure does not become less by IV mannitol, spinal drain is put in to remove enough CSF, to reduce its pressure. (Mostly it is not required.)

This will reduce the flow of perilymph and may allow the window to be sealed by a vein graft and put the prosthesis. The vein graft used here should be large enough to get good support from the surrounding tissue around the footplate. Enough pressure is exerted over the vein graft by Gelfoam packing around the piston to prevent its bulging laterally by collection of perilymph under the vein graft.

Persistent Stapedial Artery (1:5,000)

Small vessels in the stapes footplate area are very common and may not interfere with the surgery.

The persistent bigger stapedial artery runs between the two crura of the stapes and blocks the oval window. In this case, it is very difficult to remove the stapes superstructure. Similarly, it is equally difficult to make the fenestra in the stapes footplate (**Fig. 24.7**).

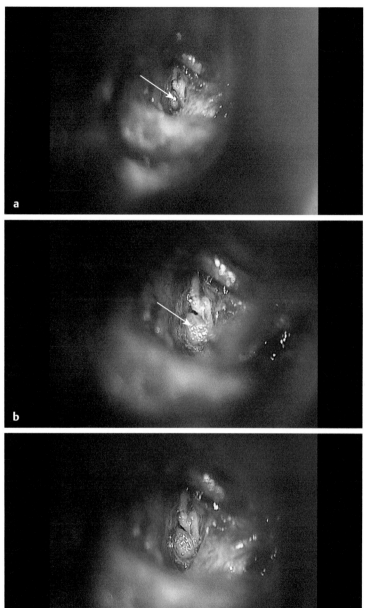

Fig. 24.6 **(a)** Part of the stapes footplate is depressed (*as shown by the arrow*) into the vestibule. **(b)** Part of the stapes footplate is depressed (*as shown by the arrow*) into the vestibule (under higher magnification). **(c)** Laser beam is focused over the depressed footplate to make a fenestra. (*Continued*)

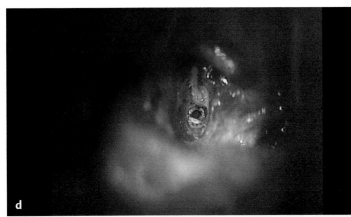

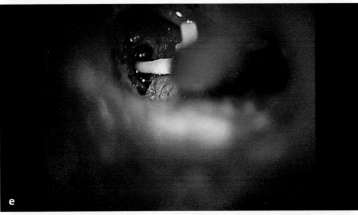

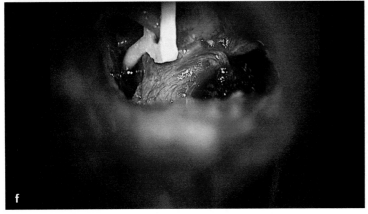

Fig. 24.6 *(Continued)* **(d)** The fenestra is made in the depressed footplate by a single shot of CO_2 laser beam. **(e)** A proper length piston is being placed between the fenestra and the incus. **(f)** A proper length piston has been placed between the fenestra and the incus. *(Continued)*

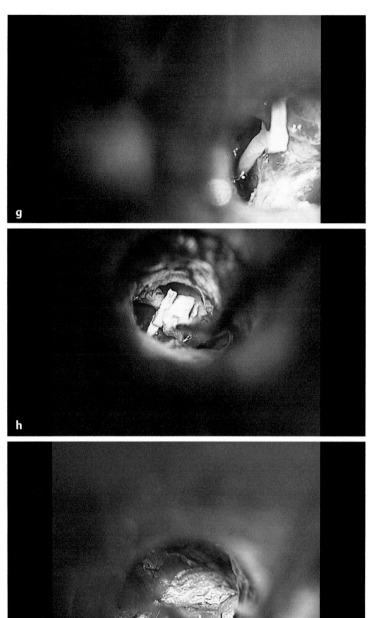

Fig. 24.6 *(Continued)* **(g)** The piston is tightened. In this patient, the lenticular process of the incus is necrosed. **(h)** The lenticular process of the incus is covered by a piece of perichondrium to prevent displacement of the piston. **(i)** The tympanomeatal flap is reposited back.

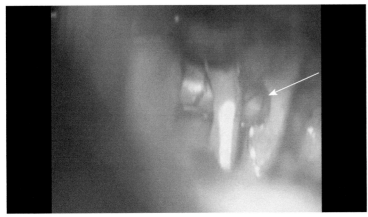

Fig. 24.7 The persistent bigger stapedial artery runs between the two crura of the stapes and blocks the oval window (*arrow*).

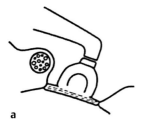
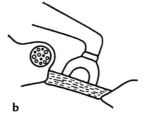
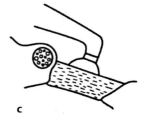

a   b   c

Fig. 24.8 (a–c) The footplate thickness in the obliterative otosclerosis varies from 0.25 to >2.50 mm.

Most of the time, the stapedial artery is anteriorly placed keeping the posterior part of the footplate available for making the fenestra. In these situations, the microdrill is the suitable tool. Use of laser is not possible here.

Big size vessel blocks the footplate completely; hence, surgery is to be abandoned.

Be careful with persistent stapedial artery as it arises from the internal carotid artery. Normally, the stapedial artery develops and degenerates during the first trimester of pregnancy.

In the author's series of 2,500 stapedectomy, there was only 1 patient of persistent stapedial artery where the procedure was abandoned.

Obliterative Otosclerosis

The disease is highly active here and the focus is highly vascular. It involves the stapes footplate and advances very fast, causing complete obliteration of the oval window and its margin. It is nothing but an advanced otosclerosis.

The process usually starts and develops around puberty and young patients in the 12- to 18-year age group are the usual patients.

In the beginning, the otosclerotic focus involves the oval window (**Fig. 24.8a**), but as the disease advances, the superstructure (crura) also gets involved (**Fig. 24.8b, c**).

Epidemiology

Incidence: Less than 5% of otosclerotic patients.

Male: The female-to-male ratio is 1.5:1. The disease is mostly bilateral.

Causes

The exact cause is not known. Various hypotheses regarding its causation are the following:

- Genetic factor.

- Immunoenzymatic process.

- Deficiency of fluoride in drinking water.

It is difficult to diagnose on the basis of clinical examination and audiogram (**Fig. 24.9**) that this otosclerotic patient is a case of obliterative otosclerosis, but certain clues will help you diagnose this condition clinically before surgery.

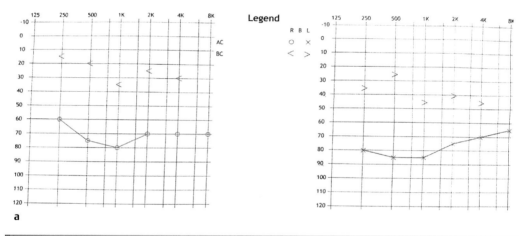

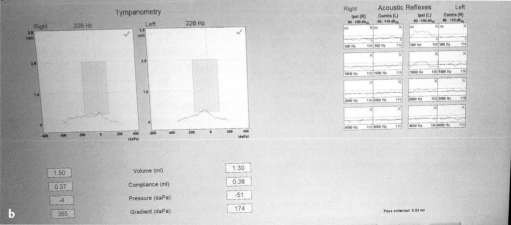

Fig. 24.9   (a) Pure tone audiogram in obliterative otosclerosis. A bilateral severe degree mixed hearing loss with an air–bone (AB) gap of 40 to 45 db. **(b)** Impedance audiogram: low compliance (As) absent stapedial reflex in both ears.

When factors like young patients coming with bilateral severe degree of conductive or mixed hearing loss, rapid progression of the disease, positive Schwartz sign, low compliance in tympanometry, and CT scan findings are present, the possibility of obliterative otosclerosis is very high.

Young patients between the ages of 12 and 20 years have a highly active otosclerotic focus (obliterative otosclerosis).

Treatment: Stapedectomy

In such young otosclerotic patients with rapid progression of the disease, medical treatment by sodium fluoride should always be started early. Sodium fluoride is given in doses of 40 mg daily along with calcium and vitamin D for a minimum of 6 months. then surgery can be performed comfortably. Sodium fluoride will slow down the disease, and difficulties during surgery are reduced by decreasing the activity and vascularity of the otosclerotic focus.

The vein graft interposition technique is contraindicated here as the active otosclerotic focus will grow fast into the mesenchymal tissues of the vein and will cause closure of the fenestra with re-fixation of the Teflon piston.

Surgery here is by the direct piston technique. The footplate fenestra made should be larger around 0.8 to 1.00 mm and the piston used is 0.4-mm thick. Extra space, which is created here around the piston, is for the new bone that is going to form postoperative due to highly active otosclerotic focus, and thus prevents re-fixation of the Teflon piston (**Fig. 24.10**).

During surgery, it is necessary to use a micro-motor or a microdrill. Drilling should be done by using diamond burr of 0.6 or 0.7 mm. Drilling should be done very slowly with intermittent pause, so that there is no heating of the bone.

Being very slow while drilling, there is no chance of damage to the facial nerve and no chance of sudden entry into the vestibule. Saucerize the entire footplate, that is, thin out the whole footplate. (Do not drill the fenestra in the footplate like a well or tunnel.) Blueline the entire footplate by a microdrill, so that a thin layer of bone covers the vestibule (**Fig. 24.11**). Now measure the distance between the footplate of the stapes and the undersurface of the long process of the incus to get an exact fit. (Measurements done before thinning the footplate are incorrect.) Then the fenestra of 0.8 mm is created in the usual way by using a pick or a perforator or by using CO_2 laser. The piston selected should be long enough not to extend more than 0.25 mm into the vestibule beyond the stapes footplate.

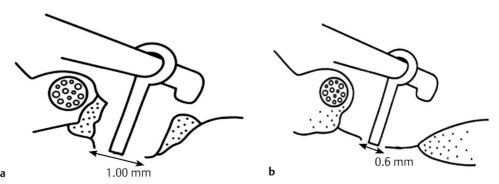

a   1.00 mm   b   0.6 mm

Fig. 24.10   **(a)** Obliterative otosclerosis, direct piston technique, fenestra is 1.00 mm and piston is 0.4 mm. In other cases fenestra is 0.6 mm and piston is 0.4 mm **(b)**.

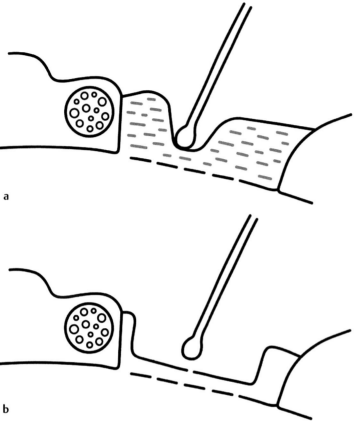

a

b

Fig. 24.11 **(a)** During surgery, it is necessary to use either a micro-motor or a microdrill. Drilling should be done by using diamond burr of 0.6 or 0.7 mm. **(b)** Saucerize the entire foot-plate, that is, thin out the whole footplate. (Do not drill the fenestra in the footplate like a well or a tunnel). Blueline the entire footplate by the microdrill, so that a thin layer of bone covers the vestibule.

A 0.4-mm-thick piston of proper length is placed and tightened, and the tympanomeatal (TM) flap is reposited (**Fig. 24.12**).

In these cases of obliterative otosclerosis, sodium fluoride should always be given postoperatively in doses of 40 mg daily for 2 years.

This will reduce the activity of the otosclerotic focus and thus decrease the chances of re-closure of the fenestra by a new bone formation.

Re-closure usually occurs within 1 year after surgery, depending upon the activity of the otosclerotic focus. Cases of re-closure can be treated by a careful revision surgery by an experienced surgeon, but results are doubtful and there is high possibility of getting SNHL. Thus, hearing aid can be given to these patients.

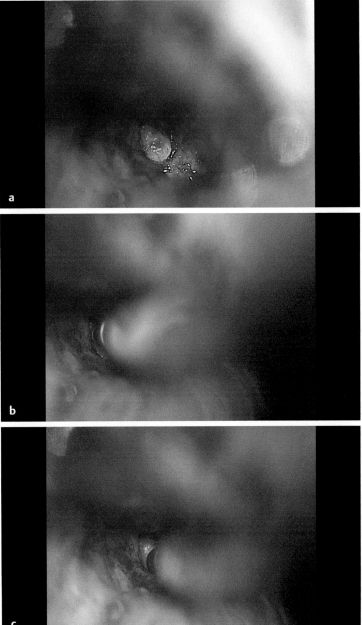

Fig. 24.12 **(a)** Thick obliterative footplate, superstructure removed. **(b, c)** The microdrill is used to thin out and saucerize the obliterative footplate. *(Continued)*

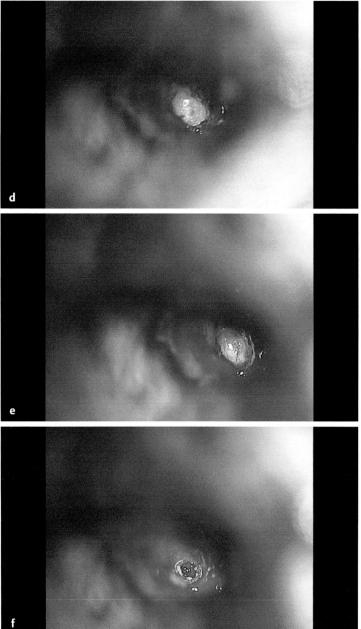

Fig. 24.12 *(Continued)* **(d)** The footplate is saucerized and *bluelined*. **(e)** CO_2 laser beam focused over the thinned out footplate. **(f)** A 0.8-mm fenestra is made in the footplate by CO_2 laser. *(Continued)*

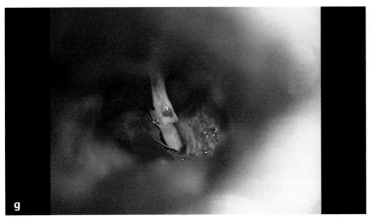

Fig. 24.12 *(Continued)* **(g)** A 0.4-mm piston of proper length is placed.

Malleus Head Fixation Combined with Otosclerosis

This should not be missed during primary surgery. the mobility of all the ossicles should be checked one by one before proceeding for stapedectomy.

Minor fixation of the head of the malleus could be due to hyalinization or calcification of the anterior mallear ligament. This can be freed by exposing, releasing, and cutting the anterior mallear ligament, and gentle pressure is exerted over the malleus, thus mobilizing it (**Fig. 24.13**).

Occasionally, the head of the malleus is fixed in the attic. this could be either due to calcification or ossification.

It is found that there is higher incidence of hyalinization of the anterior mallear ligament and higher incidence of bony fixation of the head of the malleus to the lateral attic wall in cases of otosclerosis.

Surgery for Malleus Head Fixation in the Attic

Here the incision is converted into endaural from endomeatal, which has been taken earlier at the start of the surgery. After elevating the TM flap, an anterior atticotomy is done by removing the lateral attic wall. The head of the malleus is freed by drilling the bone that is fixing it by using diamond bur of 1 mm. Gelfilm or Silastic is placed between the head of the malleus and the attic wall to prevent future adhesions and the atticotomy is closed by a cartilage. Stapedectomy is performed at the same time.

Malleus head fixation in the attic may be associated with fixation of the body of the incus in the attic due to ossification. This can also be treated simultaneously in a similar manner by doing anterior atticotomy, drilling out the bone-fixing incus, and closing the attic defect by cartilage after keeping a gelfilm between the incus body and the attic wall to prevent future adhesions.

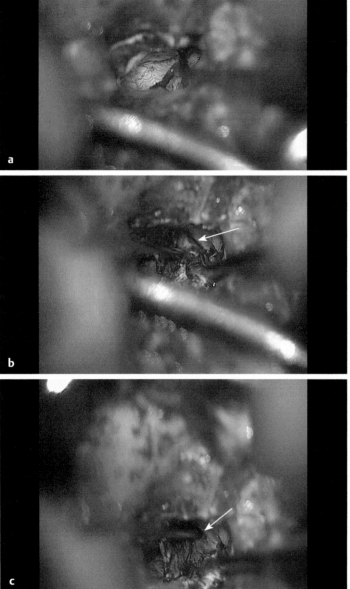

Fig. 24.13 (a) Checking the mobility of all the ossicles one by one before proceeding for stapedectomy. **(b)** Minor fixation of the malleus could be due to hyalinization or calcification of the anterior mallear ligament. The *arrow* shows the anterior mallear ligament (*arrow*). **(c)** The malleus can be freed by exposing, releasing, and stretching the anterior mallear ligament (*arrow*). *(Continued)*

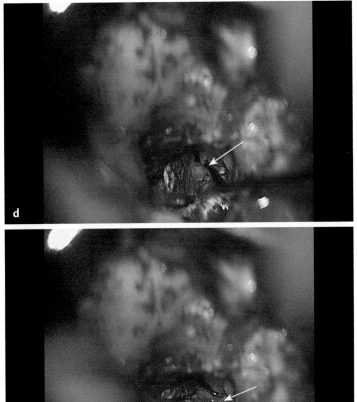

Fig. 24.13 *(Continued)* **(d)** If required, the malleus is freed by exposing and cutting the anterior mallear ligament *(arrow)*. **(e)** The malleus got mobilized by cutting the anterior mallear ligament with gentle pressure exerted over the malleus handle *(arrow)*.

Severe degree of fixation of the malleus head can be treated by removal of the malleus head by a malleus head nipper, followed by malleostapedotomy by putting a piston between the handle of the malleus and the footplate fenestra (**Fig. 24.14**).

Incus Bypass Technique

When the middle ear is opened for stapedectomy, one of the following can appear:

- The lenticular process of the incus is found to be necrosed or the incus

is found to be completely destroyed (**Fig. 24.15a**).

- Occasionally, the incus lenticular process is found to be short and it is not possible to put the piston between the footplate fenestra and the incus, especially when the fallopian canal is dehiscent and the facial nerve is bulging.

- At times, the incus is missing, which could be dislocated by the previous surgeon in cases of revision surgeries (**Fig. 24.15b**).

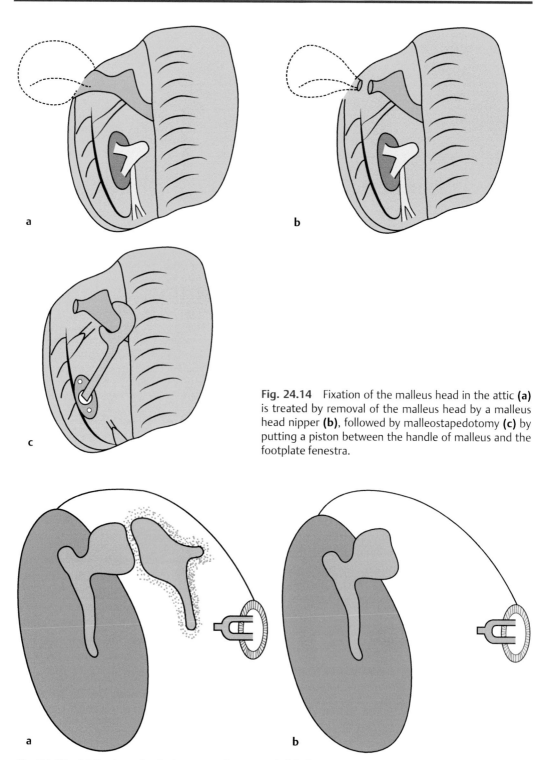

Fig. 24.14   Fixation of the malleus head in the attic **(a)** is treated by removal of the malleus head by a malleus head nipper **(b)**, followed by malleostapedotomy **(c)** by putting a piston between the handle of malleus and the footplate fenestra.

Fig. 24.15   (a) The incus lenticular process is necrosed. **(b)** The incus is missing.

Various incus bypass techniques are required here. For overall incus problem, various alternative arrangements are the following:

- Malleus to footplate teflon piston (malleostapedotomy; **Fig. 24.16a**).

- Cartilage on vein graft (Dr. A. B. R. Desai's technique).

Malleus to Footplate Teflon Piston

The advantage in this arrangement is that the malleus to footplate piston is readily available.

However, there are two disadvantages of this arrangement:

- The piston here is not exactly at right angle to the footplate fenestra. The piston is oblique here because the malleus is anterior to the stapes footplate in the middle ear; hence, effective sound transmission is not there.

- It is not easy to fit the piston between the malleus handle and the stapes footplate fenestra, especially when the malleus is very much anterior to the stapes.

Both these problems can be taken care of by specially designed titanium prosthesis.

- Chances of extrusion of the piston are very high, as the piston loop is very close to the tympanic membrane. This extrusion can be avoided by placing a very small piece of perichondrium or vein graft lateral to the piston loop at the handle of the malleus so that there will be no contact between the piston and the drum.

- Chances of damage to the oval window membrane by the movement of the piston are very high, because the piston moves in and out with the movement of the malleus handle while cleaning the ear and may cause permanent SNHL.

This can be minimized by the following:

- Placing the piston over the handle of the malleus very close to the lateral process of the malleus where the lateral movement of the malleus handle is minimum.

- By covering the stapes footplate fenestra by the vein graft before placing the piston.

By using a ball and socket titanium prosthesis.

Cartilage on Vein Graft (Dr. A. B. R. Desai's Technique)

Here the tragal cartilage is used in place of prosthesis. A bigger size fenestra is made in the footplate of the stapes. it is then covered by a bigger size vein graft with the intima facing the middle ear and a **Y**-shaped cartilage is placed between the malleus handle and the footplate fenestra which is covered by a vein graft (**Fig. 24.16b**).

There are two types of arrangements:

- If the incus is absent or its long process is very much destroyed, cartilage is kept between the malleus handle and the footplate fenestra, covered by a vein graft.

- If the sufficient length of the long process of the incus is present (only the lenticular process is destroyed), cartilage is kept between the long process of the incus and the footplate fenestra, covered by a vein graft.

Advantages:

- This is the best and safest technique as the cartilage is a very soft and

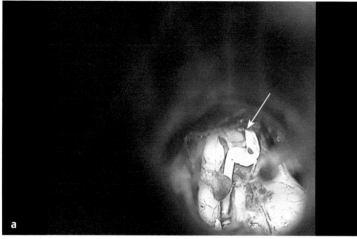

Fig. 24.16 (a) Malleostapedotomy for a short incus. The *arrow* shows a piston attached to the malleus handle just below the lateral process of the malleus with its lower end in the footplate fenestra. (b) A Y-shaped cartilage is placed between the malleus handle and the footplate fenestra which is covered by the vein graft.

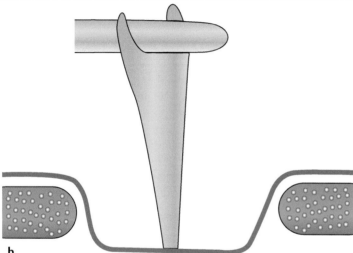

elastic structure and will not perforate the vein graft or the oval window membrane. hence, there is no chance of any trauma to the inner ear.

- Easily available.
- No cost.

Short Incus

An otosclerotic patient having a short incus lenticular process with or without a dehiscent fallopian canal is not uncommon. here, it is not possible to place the teflon piston between the incus and the footplate fenestra. In addition, at times the oval window slit is deep and narrow due to a bulging promontory and a fallopian canal causing additional difficulty while placing the piston (**Fig. 24.17**).

The best alternative is to place the piston between the malleus handle and the footplate fenestra covered by a vein graft (malleostapedotomy).

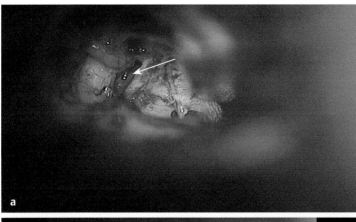

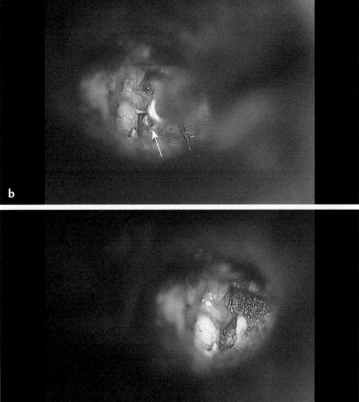

Fig. 24.17 **(a)** The middle ear exposed. Narrow and deep oval window slit, bulging facial nerve, prominent and bulging promontory, and short incus shown by *arrow*. **(b)** Prominent and bulging promontory hiding the stapes footplate drilled by a microdrill (*arrow*). **(c)** Adequate stapes footplate exposed after drilling the promontory margin. *(Continued)*

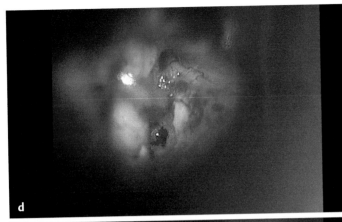

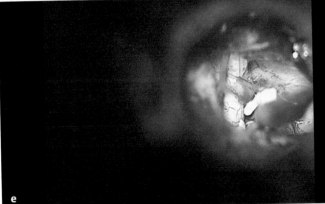

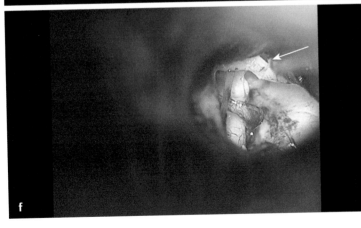

Fig. 24.17 *(Continued)* **(d)** Very good exposure of the stapes footplate after drilling the bulging promontory. A 1-mm fenestra is made in the stapes footplate by a microdrill. **(e)** Attempt was made to place the Teflon piston between the incus and the footplate fenestra, but it was not possible due to short lenticular process of the incus and bulging facial nerve. **(f)** A tunnel is made between the tympanic membrane and the handle of malleus (*arrow*) by incising the periosteum of handle of the malleus just below the lateral process of the malleus for placement of a Teflon piston (malleostapedotomy). *(Continued)*

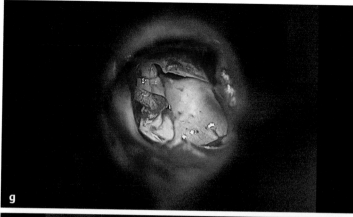

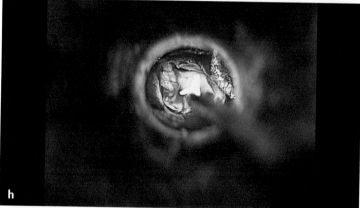

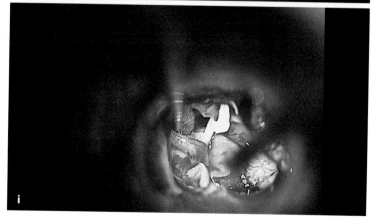

Fig. 24.17 *(Continued)* **(g)** The footplate fenestra is covered by the vein graft with the intima facing the middle ear. **(h, i)** The Teflon piston is placed between the malleus handle and the footplate fenestra covered by the vein graft. Mobile short incus and malleus head is not removed as it is not affecting the ultimate outcome of the surgery. *(Continued)*

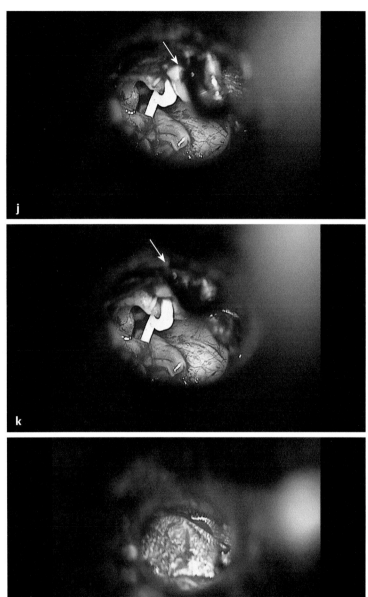

Fig. 24.17 *(Continued)* **(j, k)** A small piece of vein graft is placed in the tunnel made between the malleus handle and the tympanic membrane lateral to the piston loop to prevent its extrusion (*arrows*). **(l)** The tympanomeatal (TM) flap is reposited back. On table hearing was satisfactory.

In patients with a short incus, the other alternative is to use Robinson bucket handle prosthesis attached to the tip of the lenticular process of the incus with a vein graft interposition to get a proper fit, maintaining a perfect 90-degree angle between the footplate fenestra and the prosthesis.

The other alternative is to use a metallic piston, which can be bent as per the need to maintain perpendicularity with the footplate.

Deep Oval Window Niche

At times, the oval window niche is very deep and narrow. the footplate is very deep due to the following:

- Bulging overhanging promontory.

- Bulging fallopian canal.

The oval window looks like a slitlike opening in the depth.

The bulging, overhanging bone of the promontory around the stapes footplate, which is hiding the footplate, is reduced with due care by a microdrill or a micromotor with diamond burr so that the whole footplate is exposed before making a fenestra in the footplate (**Fig. 24.18**).

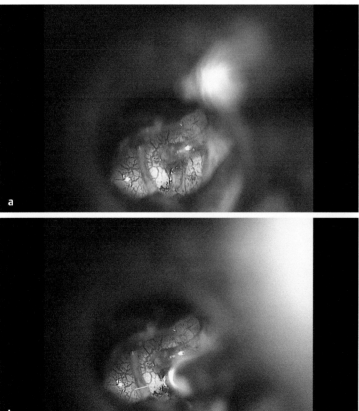

Fig. 24.18 (a) Deep oval window niche due to the bulging promontory and bulging fallopian canal. (b) The bulging promontory is reduced by a microdrill with diamond bur of 1.00 mm (*arrow*). (*Continued*)

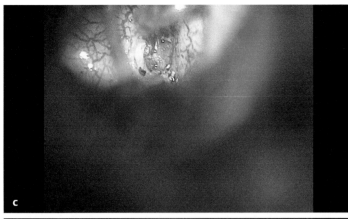

Fig. 24.18 *(Continued)* **(c)** After drilling the promontory, sufficient footplate has been exposed to make the fenestra. **(d)** A 0.6-mm fenestra is made in the footplate by CO_2 laser. **(e)** A 0.4-mm piston is placed between the incus and the footplate fenestra. The piston is then tightened and the tympanomeatal (TM) flap is reposited.

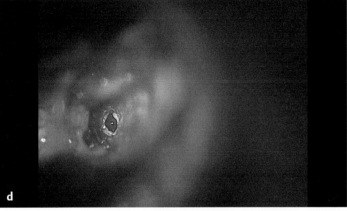

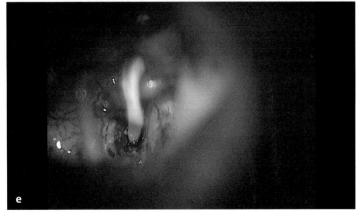

25 Operation in the Second Ear

Operation in the second ear should only be planned after a gap of 1 year after the first ear surgery, as there is always a possibility of delayed sensorineural hearing loss (SNHL) after stapes surgery.

Surgery of the second ear should only be planned if the first ear surgery is successful, there is good closure of the air–bone gap, and the patient does not experience vertigo.

However, there are certain contraindications to operation in the second ear, some of which are the following:

- If the surgery in the first ear was difficult and eventful.

- If the patient develops some complications like vertigo and SNHL following surgery in the first ear.

- Certain people are not in favor of performing surgery in the second ear as they do not want to expose both the ears to the possibility of delayed SNHL after surgery.

26 Revision Stapedectomy

Introduction

The need for a revision surgery arises under the following circumstances:

- When the patient says that there is no improvement in the hearing following the first surgery.

- When the patient says that there was an improvement in the hearing following surgery in the beginning, which lasted only for a few days to months, followed by decreased hearing.

- Worsening of hearing following stapedectomy usually associated with vertigo which is severe at times. The deafness may be fluctuating sometimes.

When investigated, the deafness in the categories 1 and 2 is mostly found to be conductive in nature and there is no need to hurry in revising these cases.

Deafness in category 3 is found to be sensorineural and early intervention is needed to prevent further and permanent damage.

It is important to remember the following facts:

- The revision surgery is more difficult than the first surgery.

- The revision surgery is not as successful as the first surgery.

- Prosthesis (Teflon piston), which has been inserted in the first surgery is in very close contact with the utricle and the saccule, with the possibility of adhesions between them. If this prosthesis is pulled blindly, there is a possibility of damage to the utricle and saccule, leading to deaf ear.

The decision of a revision stapedectomy should be taken carefully because of the following reasons:

- As mentioned earlier, the revision surgery is not safe and not as successful as the primary surgery.

- There are varieties of situations, which are faced during the revision surgery, which affects the ultimate outcome.

- There are more chances of getting sensorineural hearing loss (SNHL) following revision surgery and high chances of nonclosure of the air–bone (AB) gap after revision stapes surgery.

Before revision surgery is planned, good hearing assessment, including fresh audiogram with perfect masking, should be done.

Undiagnosed unilateral SNHL in the operated ear with false-negative Rinne test should always be ruled out, which might have been missed before the first surgery. Proper Rinne and Weber tests should be done to confirm SNHL in the ear to be operated on.

A review of the audiogram conducted before the first surgery should always be done, which at times is confusing. A fresh audiogram with proper masking should be done.

The surgeon, if he is revising his own case, if possible, should try to recollect all the steps of the surgery that he has performed. He will definitely be able to recollect and point out where things went wrong. If the procedure has been recorded, then the surgeon can review the recordings and find out the mistake, which can be corrected during the revision surgery.

If the surgery was performed by another surgeon, try to get the discharge summary and go through the operation notes, which at times are misleading. Many times, a discharge summary is not available with the patient.

High-resolution computed tomography (HRCT) of the temporal bone should be done before revising the case.

Causes of Residual or Reappearance of Conductive Hearing Loss Following Stapedectomy

Reappearance of conductive hearing loss following stapedectomy could be due to some immediate and late causes. These causes are discussed briefly in the following sections.

Immediate Causes

Immediate causes of the reappearance of conductive hearing loss include:

- **Migration or displacement of the prosthesis (piston):** This can be prevented by performing stapedotomy rather than stapedectomy, by creating a clean and discrete fenestra, putting a piston of exact length (it should neither be short nor long), and proper crimping of the piston. The length of the piston is of utmost importance.

- **Loose piston:** This could be due to improper crimping of the piston causing a gap between the incus and the piston, leading to conductive hearing loss. In few patients, the long process of the incus is thin and the piston remains loose in spite of firm crimping. This situation can be handled by using a piston with a narrow loop (e.g., Shea's piston).

- **Short piston:** This indicates that the piston is not touching the oval window membrane. Short piston is due to faulty calculation of the distance between the incus and the footplate of the stapes. It can also occur due to improper crimping of the piston. Short piston can get easily displaced while sneezing.

- **Malleus head fixation:** This was probably missed during the first surgery. Hence, the mobility of each individual ossicle should always be checked during surgery.

In addition the surgeon should also look for the following:

- Whether a round window obliteration (which is very rare) has been missed.

- Whether a superior semicircular canal dehiscence (third window) has been missed. This is again a very rare situation.

Late Causes

Reappearance of conductive hearing loss following stapedectomy could be due to:

- Displacement or migration of the prosthesis from the center of the fenestra touching the edges of the fenestra. During healing, the connective tissue seal at the fenestra, if very thick, may shrink, pushing the piston out, causing conductive hearing loss. Among all the tissue seals, the vein graft is the most suitable as it is thin and there is no chance of shrinkage.

- Fibrous adhesions may develop around the prosthesis between the incus and the promontory causes late conductive hearing loss.

- Displacement of the prosthesis from the incus, which may be complete at times.

- Incus erosion or necrosis: It is rare with teflon piston. It is common with metallic prostheses. Ideally, there should not be any movement between the incus and the loop of the prosthesis (piston). Incus necrosis usually takes place due to relative movements between the long process of the incus and the loop of the piston. this movement is due to either loose piston or tight fit of the piston in the fenestra preventing free movement of the Teflon piston in the fenestra.

Incus erosion was said to be due to decreased blood supply to the incus after section of the stapedius tendon, but it is the bone marrow in the incus that provides sufficient blood supply to the incus. Another cause for incus erosion is found to be foreign body reaction to the piston, causing local bony erosion with granulation. Clinically the incus erosion presents with the hearing loss, which is conductive in nature and fluctuates in the beginning with the head movements, but later it becomes persistent.

- Regrowth of the otosclerotic focus: It is more common with the obliterative otosclerosis. Hence, the footplate fenestra in these patients should be made much larger than the piston to prevent fixation of the piston due to new bone formation.

Surgical Steps in Revision Surgery

Revision surgery preferably should be done under local anaesthesia. The incision is either endomeatal or endaural, depending upon the surgeon and the situation. If the surgeon feels that the exposure is going to be inadequate with an endomeatal incision, then he or she should start the surgery by an endaural incision rather than struggling with inadequate exposure with the endomeatal incision, especially in a narrow external auditory canal.

Once the middle ear is entered, the first structure seen is the incus with the piston, which was placed during the previous surgery. Most of the time, the incus is covered by adhesions between the incus, tympanic membrane, and the middle ear promontory mucosa, which are to be cut either by a sickle knife or by microscopic scissors.

One must look for a loose or displaced piston.

The piston should not to be removed suddenly unless its lower end into the footplate area is defined. Usually, there are mucosal adhesions around the piston, which are to be broken and removed. CO_2 laser is very useful in performing this task atraumatically.

Examine the stapes footplate for any fenestra. if a fenestra is present in the footplate and the piston is in the fenestra, it should not to be removed. Look for round window reflex.

If round window reflex is present, the piston should not to be removed.

If round window reflex is absent, gently dissect the piston out of the fenestra, if possible by using CO_2 laser.

Palpate the malleus and incus for mobility. Check for any fixation of the malleus or incus, which might have been missed in the previous surgery.

If bony fixation of the malleus or incus is found, that should be taken care of before making a new fenestra and putting a piston.

Look for any incus erosion or necrosis. If the incus lenticular process is destroyed and is not useful, the incus is removed and malleostapedotomy can be planned.

If the malleus and the incus are normal and mobile, stapedotomy is performed.

Examine the fenestra. Get an idea about the diameter of the fenestra; if it is inadequate, it can be enlarged by microdrill or laser.

If the previous fenestra has been closed by highly active otosclerotic focus, then a new fenestra is to be made by using a microdrill and/or laser.

Get an idea about the length of the piston required by measuring the distance between the footplate and the undersurface of the incus and add 0.25 mm to it for the thickness of the footplate.

If it is not a case of obliterative otosclerosis, cover the fenestra with the vein graft and place the already-prepared piston.

In obliterative otosclerosis, the vein graft interposition technique is not done. The direct piston technique is used instead.

The tympanomeatal (TM) flap is reposited, and on table hearing is tested.

Case 1

This is a case of revision Surgery in a patient who was operated on few months back at a different center. The same ear was reexplored for persistent conductive hearing loss after the first surgery. There was no fenestra in the footplate. the footplate was obliterative, which was thinned out (saucerized) by a microdrill and the fenestra was made by CO_2 laser. A proper size piston was then placed (**Fig. 26.1**).

Recommendations for Surgeons

- For conductive hearing loss, there is no hurry. Wait for 6 to 8 months so that the middle ear mucosa comes back to normal and surgery can be performed without any difficulty.

- Avoid general anesthesia. Local anesthesia with light sedation is always preferred as under local anesthesia, if the patient experiences any vertigo on the operation table while manipulating the piston, which was placed in the previous surgery, it implies that there are adhesions between the piston and the membranous labyrinth. this is a warning for the surgeon to be cautious. In addition, hearing assessment can also be done on the operation table immediately after surgery.

- Both these assessments are not possible under general anesthesia.

- Blind manipulation of the piston, in the oval window fenestra should be avoided as that may damage the inner ear.

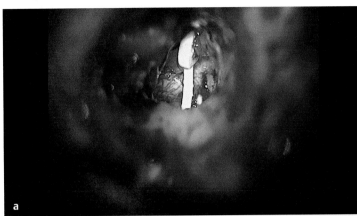

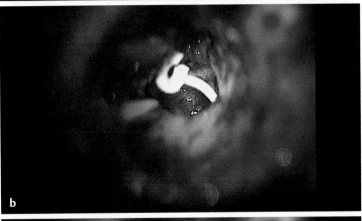

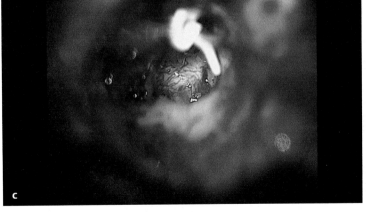

Fig. 26.1 **(a)** A case of revision surgery. On exploration, it was observed that the teflon piston was displaced laterally away from the stapes footplate but still attached to the incus. There was no stapes superstructure and no footplate fenestra. The stapes footplate was thick and obliterative. **(b)** The piston is taken out from the incus. **(c)** The piston is removed from the middle ear. No stapes super-structure is seen. *(Continued)*

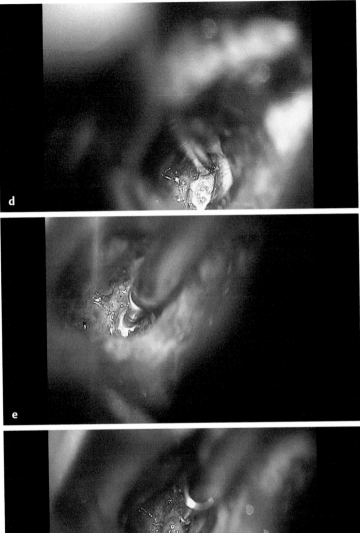

Fig. 26.1 *(Continued)* **(d)** The footplate of the stapes is exposed. It is thick and obliterative. The mobility of the incus and malleus is checked and both were found to be mobile. **(e)** The footplate of the stapes is saucerized by the microdrill with diamond bur of 0.6 mm. **(f)** Complete footplate of the stapes is thinned out uniformly and *bluelined*. *(Continued)*

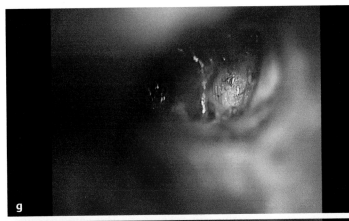

g

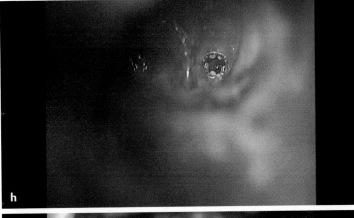

h

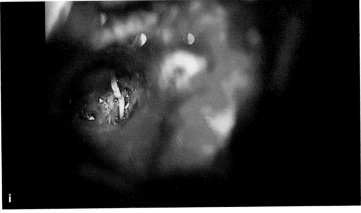

i

Fig. 26.1 *(Continued)* **(g)** CO_2 laser beam is focused over the footplate to make a fenestra. **(h)** A 0.8-mm fenestra is made by CO_2 laser in the posterior part of the footplate. A single shot is enough to make a discrete fenestra in the stapes footplate. **(i)** A 0.4-mm piston of suitable length is placed between the incus and the footplate fenestra by the direct piston technique. The tympanomeatal (TM) flap is reposited back after crimping the piston.

- If the surgeon is not able to find any fault during the revision surgery, he or she should close the middle ear.

- CO_2 laser is very useful during the revision surgery. The introduction of laser for revision stapedectomy has improved the hearing results.

- A rare but undoubtedly an important point of consideration is that obliteration of the round window by the otosclerotic focus should always be kept in mind and its patency should always be checked during the primary surgery.

Results

Results of revision surgeries are not as good as those of primary surgeries. A revision surgery provides a good closure of the AB gap in more than 75% of cases with a little more risk of SNHL following the surgery than the primary surgery.

There are less chances of complete closure of the AB gap in a revision surgery as compared to the primary surgery and some AB gap (around 30 dB) remains in spite of a good uneventful surgery. The reason for this is not known.

There are more chances of developing SNHL in the revision surgery as compared to the primary surgery. This could be due to trauma to the inner ear and blind manipulations in the area of the footplate fenestra. Hence, it is essential to be careful before taking the decision to perform a revision stapedectomy. Using CO_2 Laser in revision surgery is advisable as it has been found to provide better results.

27 Perilymph Fistula

Introduction

This is the most preventable cause of sensorineural hearing loss (SNHL) following stapedectomy. The fistula may be primary or secondary. The primary fistula is formed the moment the fenestra is made in the footplate; gradually, the oval window membrane is formed and the fistula closes. The secondary fistula develops later, may be days or months after stapedectomy.

If the oval window membrane (endosteal membrane) is not formed or it is ruptured due to some reason, then there will be possibility of the formation of a perilymph fistula. Fistulas may be early or late in development.

The causes for the formation of perilymph fistula are the following:

- Early fistulas are due to failure of formation of the oval window membrane, which could be due to the following:
  - Long piston.
  - Large fenestra.
- Late fistulas are due to rupture of the already formed oval window membrane, which could be due to the following:
  - The piston is pulled in to the vestibule:
    - By the negative middle ear pressure due to eustachian tube (ET) block.
    - Or due to formation of adhesions from the lenticular process of the incus to raw promontory, which develops gradually, pulling the piston medially.
  - The piston is pushed in by acoustic trauma or barotrauma (mountaineering, flying).
  - If positive pressure is exerted over the tympanic membrane it will cause displacement of piston in to the vestibule causing SNHL.

Remember that covering the fenestra by the vein graft before putting the piston will not prevent development of a perilymph fistula as the leak is always submucosal and if the piston is long, it will perforate the vein graft.

Diagnosis

After an initial improvement in the hearing, there is a fluctuating deafness associated with fullness in the ear, tinnitus, and vertigo, which may be mild to severe (symptoms are like Meniere's disease).

Audiogram shows that bone conduction of the operated ear has fallen below that of the unoperated ear, after initial improvement, giving rise to a mixed variety of hearing loss.

Fistula test by pneumatic otoscope is negative in most of the patients, but fistula test with electronystagmography (ENG) is very reliable in diagnosis of perilymph fistula.

Management

As it is mentioned earlier that this is the most preventable cause of sensorineural hearing loss following Stapedectomy. Perilymph fistula can be avoided by creating a discrete fenestra of 0.6 mm with piston of 0.4 mm of perfect length with perfect crimping of piston. Postoperatively these patient should avoid straining, coughing, lifting heavy weights, and barotrauma.

Once the perilymph fistula is suspected, the ear should be explored as early as possible, to prevent further deterioration of hearing. Treatment is to close the fistula by surgery.

When the surgery is performed and the ear is explored, it is not easy to diagnose the perilymph fistula, as there is no free flow of fluid in to the middle ear like cerebrospinal fluid (CSF) otorrhea or gusher. Fluid is in microliter and it is very difficult to see the leak. Under higher magnification, you can see the drop of perilymph leaking from the oval window area, after mopping the area by dry gelfoam.

Expose the area nicely; if necessary, dissect the piston from the oval window membrane at the footplate fenestra and remove it under direct vision.

Examine the fenestra; if it is adequate, cover it by a vein graft and put a piston of proper size.

CO_2 laser is very much useful in managing these cases. It is also very useful in breaking the adhesions, dissecting the tissues at the oval window fenestra before removal of piston, and in making a new fenestra in the oval window.

If, on exploration, the surgeon is not able to find any leak, the best thing is to remove the piston with due care, make a discrete fenestra of 0.8 mm (if the earlier fenestra is not proper), cover it with the vein graft, and put a piston of 0.4 mm thickness of suitable length.

Usually prognosis is good in these cases, if explored early.

28 Far-Advanced Otosclerosis

Introduction

Far-advanced otosclerosis (FAO) is defined as when there is no recordable air and bone conduction. Air conduction (AC) is more than 95 dB and bone conduction (BC) is more than 55 dB and is not recordable by pure tone audiometers.

Profound hearing loss but negative Rinne test at 256 Hz indicates FAO. While doing an audiogram, always do BC at 3,000 Hz. At other frequencies, no BC is recordable. Recordable BC may be present at 3,000 Hz in cases of advanced otosclerosis.

In otosclerosis, BC at 2,000 Hz is not recordable at times due to carhart notch and BC at 4,000 Hz is not recordable due to presbyacusis in older people.

Diagnosis

Well-modulated voice, family history of otosclerosis, tuning fork test, audiometry, and high-resolution computed tomography (HRCT) of the temporal bones will help in diagnosis of advanced otosclerosis.

CT scan of the temporal bone shows disease severity and helps grade the advanced otosclerosis.

On CT scan, presence of pericochlear lucency is specific for cochlear otosclerosis.

Magnetic resonance imaging (MRI) show a ring with an intermediate signal and is usually detected in the pericochlear area, which is specific for cochlear otosclerosis. MRI can also detect cochlear duct patency.

Kabbara classified advanced otosclerosis into three stages based on the CT scan of the temporal bone:

- Stage 1: Lesion is characterized by limited footplate involvement with pericochlear lesion without endosteum involvement.

- Stage 2: Lesion with significant pericochlear and endosteal involvement.

- Stage 3: Lesion is characterized by full obliteration of the round window and/or basal turn ossification with pericochlear lesion.

Another classification is by Rotteveel:

- Type 1: Solely fenestral involvement.

- Type 2: Retrofenestral with or without fenestral involvement.

- Type 2a: Double-ring effect.

- Type 2b: Narrowed basal turn.

- Type 2c: Double-ring effect and narrowed basal turn.

- Type 3: Severe retrofenestral with or without fenestral involvement (unrecognizable otic capsule).

Treatment

The treatment options for FAO are the following:

- Hearing aid without surgery, if useful.

- Salvage surgery (stapedectomy) with hearing aid. Here the patient should be selected with significant conductive component (significant air–bone gap) with a good speech discrimination score. Patients with more than 50% discrimination scores are associated with better results.

- There were patients who were candidates for cochlear implant (CI) but had undergone stapedectomy and were able to use a hearing aid after surgery with good results. Studies have shown around 80% of such patients were satisfied by surgery and could use hearing aids after stapedectomy with good results. Hence, stapedectomy should always be performed before considering them for CI.

- In patients with failed stapedectomy, CI should be done.

- CI should always be done in patients with poor speech discrimination score (<30%), with poor hearing aid outcome, and in patients having small AB gap. These patients should go for primary CI rather than going for stapedectomy first.

CI is very useful, but difficulty during electrode insertion may be there due to sclerosis. Kabbara stage 1 and 2 advanced otosclerosis are easy to implant. In Kabbara stage 3, where there is ossification in the basal turn of the cochlea, it is difficult to implant.

29 Otosclerosis and Pregnancy

Many times, an otosclerotic patient says that the deafness started during pregnancy.

Certain patients say that deafness increased during pregnancy.

It is not true in all the cases. It is found that repeated pregnancy in few otosclerotic patients did not worsen their hearing.

The increased estrogen level in the body during pregnancy causes release of certain lysosomal enzymes that activate the otosclerotic focus.

It is found that in pregnancy, following stapedectomy in one ear, hearing loss progressed more in the nonoperated ear as compared to the operated ear.

This shows that stapedectomy gives some protection from further hearing loss in the operated ear during pregnancy following surgery.

30 Stapedectomy and Air Travel

In the direct piston technique, in which the vein graft is not used to cover the footplate fenestra, healing takes place slowly and oval window membrane is formed gradually. The tissues at the fenestra are infiltrated by polymorphs within 24 hours. These polymorphs are then replaced by fibroblasts within 48 hours. Thin membrane of fibrocytes forms within 1 week. By 3 weeks, a firm fibrous membrane is formed.

Hence, these 3 weeks are very crucial, and the patient should take all possible precautions during these 3 weeks. Hence, air travel should not be permitted at least for 3 weeks following surgery.

Comparatively air travel is safer when the window is sealed by the vein graft.

Overall air travel is relatively safe following stapedectomy, provided the eustachian tube (ET) function is normal and there is no upper respiratory tract infection (URI) causing ET block.

Similarly scuba diving is not risky if the ET is functioning well. However, it is safer when the window is sealed by the vein graft.

31 Sensorineural Hearing Loss Following Stapedectomy

Introduction

Sensorineural hearing loss (SNHL) is the most dangerous complication of a stapes surgery. It may be sudden or gradual. It may be temporary or permanent. Incidence of SNHL following stapedectomy is around 1 to 3%. It may be mild to total hearing loss. It can also be selective SNHL for high frequency.

The development of this complication depends upon the surgeon's experience and the disease process including cochlear involvement.

All the patients should be informed about this complication before surgery.

SNHL may be "sudden" due to loss of the perilymph, which is either due to perilymph gusher or due to accidental suction by the surgeon, near the oval window fenestra. Sometimes it is due to associated hydrops leading to sudden loss of perilymph after making the fenestra.

SNHL may be "gradual" due to perilymph fistula. Hearing loss in these cases is fluctuating many a times.

Causes of Temporary SNHL

- *Serous labyrinthitis:* It is nothing but labyrinthine reaction to surgical manipulations in the stapes footplate area associated with vertigo of mild to moderate degree and lasts for 1 or 2 days. This labyrinthine reaction resolves quickly with symptomatic treatment without any sequelae.

- *Reparative granuloma:* Granuloma formation in the footplate area is not very common and usually develops a week after surgery and is associated with pain in the ear due to middle ear involvement with SNHL and vertigo if it enters the vestibule. Usually it is said to be a reaction to some foreign body like cotton fiber or gelfoam or fat.

Clinically, the eardrum is congested and thickened especially in its posterosuperior part.

Audiogram shows mixed hearing loss (both conductive and sensorineural) with poor speech discrimination score (<50%).

Treatment of Reparative Granuloma

These cases should be explored immediately (within 15 days of onset of symptoms). then, the chances of recovery are high. Hearing comes back to near normal and there is no residual SNHL.

Surgery involves exploratory tympanotomy. The granuloma should be dissected nicely and excised with complete removal. If required, the piston is to be removed with due care and a new piston should be placed after removing the granuloma. Immediate diagnosis and prompt action is always fruitful. Good antibiotics and steroids are to be given both intraoperatively and postoperatively.

Causes of Permanent SNHL

- It occurs as a result of traumatic and clumsy footplate surgery while making the fenestra or while making attempts to remove a footplate bone piece from the vestibule especially in cases of a depressed footplate causing rupture of the basilar membrane.

- It can also occur due to a sudden drop in the perilymph pressure due to use of suction near the footplate fenestra causing rupture of the Reissner membrane.

- Ganglion cells of the inner ear can be damaged by normal saline or Ringer's lactate entering the inner ear causing SNHL.

Treatment

Full care should be taken to prevent SNHL. If it occurs, intravenous (IV) steroids are given. Hydrocortisone is preferred in high doses and repeated every 6 hours. High doses of methyl prednisolone are also a good alternative to hydrocortisone.

Nicotinic acid injection should be given IV every 6 hours. It is used as a vasodilator.

IV heparin is also administered to improve blood circulation.

This treatment is to be continued for at least 1 week, followed by oral steroids.

It is very difficult to predict ultimate outcome in these patients and SNHL of mild to severe degree may be the end result. This complication following stapes surgery is like a nightmare and full care should be taken to prevent it.

32 Indications for Hearing Aid in Otosclerosis

Introduction

Patients who have been advised surgery should always be told about the alternatives to surgery, that is, nothing but hearing aid. Otherwise hearing aid should always be given to the following:

- Patients not willing to undergo surgery or those unfit for surgery.

- Patients with only one hearing ear. The other ear is dead either due to an unsuccessful surgery or due to disease.

- Patients having poor cochlear function or poor speech discrimination score. Surgery in these cases is not very fruitful. Hearing aid can be tried in these patients.

- Patients having both otosclerosis and endolymphatic hydrops.

- Patients with congenital fixation of stapes. The disease is nonprogressive and there are more chances of perilymph gusher and sensorineural hearing loss (SNHL) in these patients.

Bone-Anchored Hearing Aids for Otosclerotic Patients

Bone-anchored hearing aids (BAHA) are a very good alternative for only hearing ear with advanced disease where the conventional hearing aid is not very useful. The main advantage of using BAHA is that there is no risk of dead ear following insertion of BAHA, which is very much there with stapedectomy. In addition, the sound quality with BAHA is better than that in conventional hearing aids. The only problem is cost. The BAHA are costly.

33 Laser Stapedotomy

Introduction

Use of laser in stapedotomy is a big landmark in the history of stapedectomy. The conventional technique of stapes surgery involves using various picks and perforators. This surgical technique is crude and risky.

Introduction of microdrill has made stapedectomy safer and simpler than the conventional technique.

Laser is a new addition in stapedectomy tool, which has made stapes surgery most convenient and safe.

Various surgeons have shown that laser can handle various difficult situations in stapedectomy easily and has made stapedectomy less complicated.

The use of laser in stapes surgery has improved the hearing results.

There is less occurrence of vertigo after surgery and thus shorter hospital stay.

Fig. 33.1 shows a laser machine being activated. **Fig. 33.2** shows a micromanipulator and how the micromanipulator is attached to the laser machine, with the laser beam coming out of the micromanipulator.

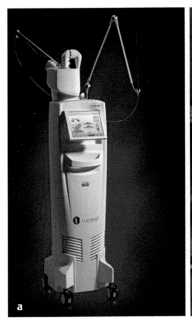
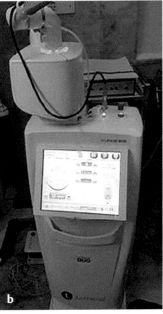

Fig. 33.1 **(a)** CO_2 laser machine. **(b)** CO_2 laser machine activated.

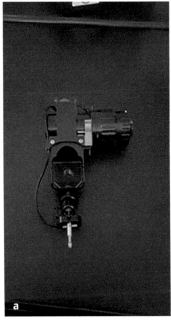
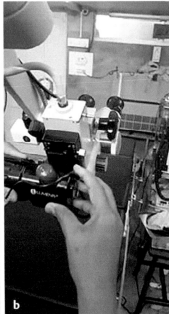
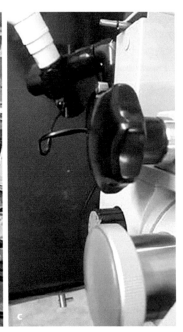

Fig. 33.2 **(a)** Micromanipulator. **(b)** Attaching the micromanipulator to the microscope. **(c)** Laser beam coming out through the micromanipulator and is controlled by joystick.

Types of Laser

There are two types of lasers, which differ from each other depending upon the lasing medium being used. These are the following:

- Visible lasers: Argon and KTP (potassium titanyl phosphate).
- Invisible laser: CO_2 laser.

Visible lasers (argon and KTP) are only absorbed by colored tissues and reflected by the white bone and the collagen of the stapes. Hence, they are not very useful in stapedotomy. A much higher laser energy is required to ablate the bone with argon and KTP lasers as compared to CO_2 laser.

CO_2 laser has ideal tissue absorption quality because this laser is absorbed by water and water content of the bone is very high. Hence, all the energy is absorbed by the footplate bone while making the fenestra before it penetrates the saccule, which makes it very safe for the vestibule.

The Ideal Laser for Stapedotomy

Laser beam used during stapedotomy should be very precise and specific in vaporizing the bone of the footplate while making a fenestra.

The thermal effect of the laser beam should not be deeper than the footplate. It should not heat the perilymph and should be safe for the vestibule.

Currently, CO_2 laser (long wavelength) is ideal for stapedotomy. CO_2 laser is invisible. Therefore, a separate visible coaxial light aiming laser beam (helium–neon) is needed with CO_2 laser.

Both types of laser beams have different wavelengths. Therefore, accurate and precise calibration is required while using them.

Advantages of Laser Stapedotomy

The advantages of using laser in stapedotomy are the following:

- Removal of stapes superstructure and creation of a precise fenestra in the stapes footplate is possible without handling the stapes mechanically.

- There is no trauma to the inner ear, hence there are no chances of postoperative vertigo and sensorineural hearing loss (SNHL).

- There is no chance of getting a floating footplate as the stapes is not handled mechanically.

- A good hemostasis can be achieved by using CO_2 laser in a coagulation mode to coagulate small vessels over the stapes footplate mucosa before making a fenestra.

Hence, laser is very much useful in both primary and revision stapedectomy.

Problems with Conventional (Mechanical) Stapedotomy

Problems with the conventional technique of stapedotomy are the following:

- Fracturing the crura of the stapes, by the pressure of the right angle hook is a very crude procedure and can cause complete removal of the stapes. Removal of the stapes in toto is very dangerous and can lead to a dead ear.

- Making a fenestra in the stapes footplate by a pick or perforator exerts a lot of pressure over the footplate and may cause either subluxation of the footplate or a floating footplate.

Both these steps can be performed by CO_2 laser in a much atraumatic way without handling the stapes mechanically and thus eliminating any chance of intraoperative complications.

Laser Stapedotomy in Early Otosclerosis

Early otosclerosis is associated with an air–bone (AB) gap of around 20 db. Here, there is a minimal fixation of the stapes footplate. There are:

- More chances of the stapes getting mobilized with mechanical stapedotomy.

- More chances of removal of the stapes in toto with mechanical stapedotomy.

- More chances of the occurrence of a floating footplate with mechanical stapedotomy.

Case 1

In this situation, CO_2 laser is an ideal tool for a safe and successful surgery. The steps involved in CO_2 laser stapedotomy are depicted in **Fig. 33.3**.

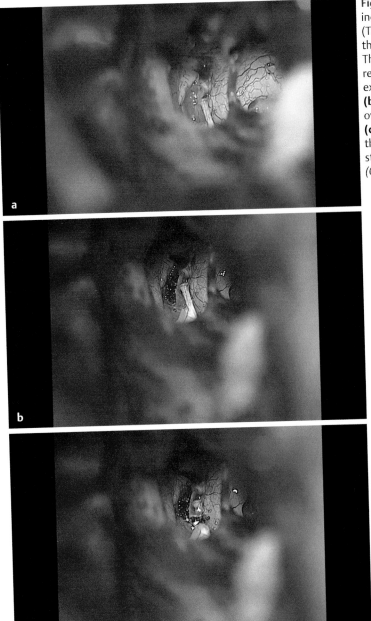

Fig. 33.3 (a) Endomeatal incision. The tympanomeatal (TM) flap is elevated and the middle ear is exposed. The meatal wall overhang is removed for getting good exposure to the stapes area. **(b)** CO_2 laser beam is focused over the stapedius muscle. **(c)** The stapedius muscle and the posterior crura of the stapes is divided by CO_2 laser. *(Continued)*

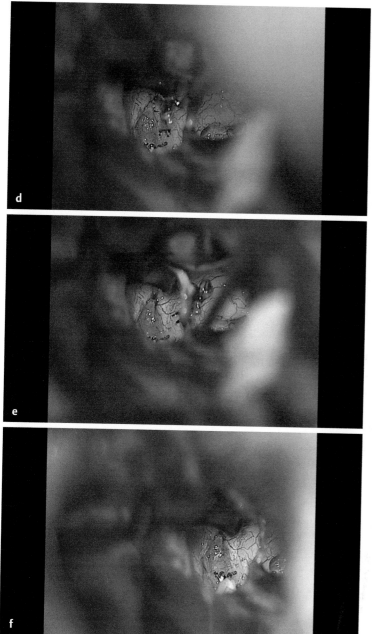

Fig. 33.3 *(Continued)* **(d)** The incudostapedial joint is separated by a right angle pick. **(e)** The stapes superstructure is removed. **(f)** Laser beam is focused over the footplate. *(Continued)*

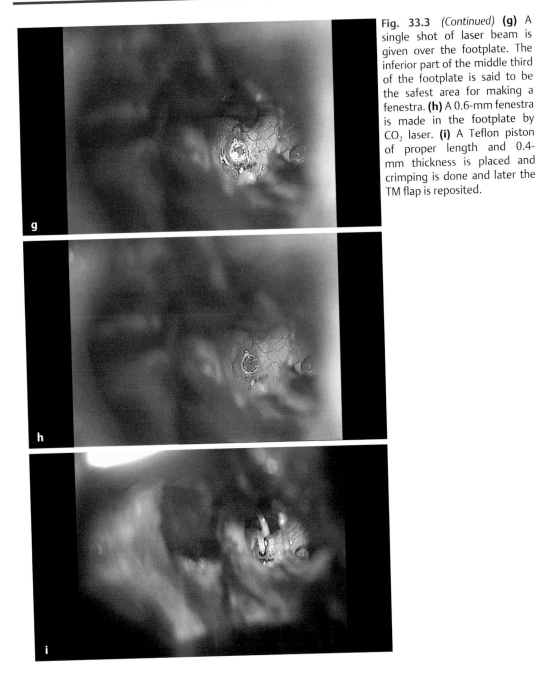

Fig. 33.3 *(Continued)* **(g)** A single shot of laser beam is given over the footplate. The inferior part of the middle third of the footplate is said to be the safest area for making a fenestra. **(h)** A 0.6-mm fenestra is made in the footplate by CO_2 laser. **(i)** A Teflon piston of proper length and 0.4-mm thickness is placed and crimping is done and later the TM flap is reposited.

Two cases of obliterative otosclerosis are briefly described in the following sections.

Case 2

In this case, surgery was performed with a microdrill and laser. It began with an endomeatal incision, followed by elevation of the tympanomeatal (TM) flap. Overhang was removed. A thick obliterative otosclerotic footplate was found. The malleus and the Incus were mobile. The footplate was thinned out by drilling it using a microdrill with diamond burr of 0.6 mm (**Fig. 33.4**).

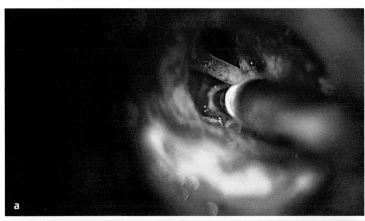

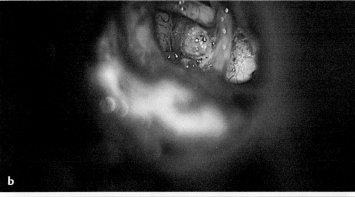

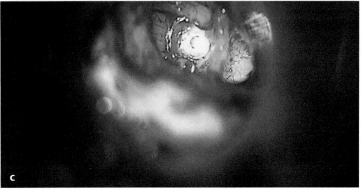

Fig. 33.4 (a) The footplate is thinned out by drilling it by using a microdrill with diamond burr of 0.6-mm thickness. The aim is to saucerize the footplate. **(b)** The footplate is blue lined. Laser beam is focused over the footplate. **(c)** A single shot of CO_2 laser beam is made on the stapes footplate. *(Continued)*

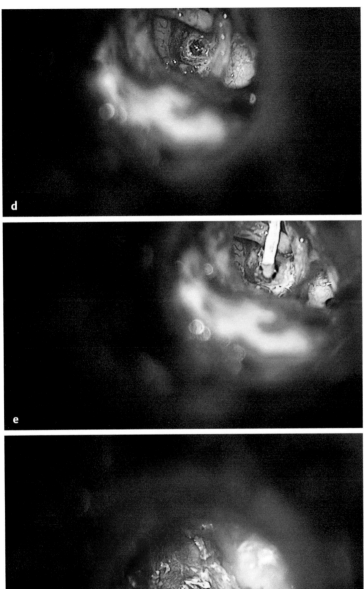

d

e

f

Fig. 33.4 *(Continued)* **(d)** A 0.6-mm fenestra is made in the footplate by CO_2 laser. **(e)** A Teflon piston of suitable length and 0.4-mm thickness is placed and tightened by crimping. **(f)** The tympanomeatal (TM) flap is reposited.

Case 3

This is a case of otosclerosis where both the anterior and posterior crura were seen and could be laserized (**Fig. 33.5**).

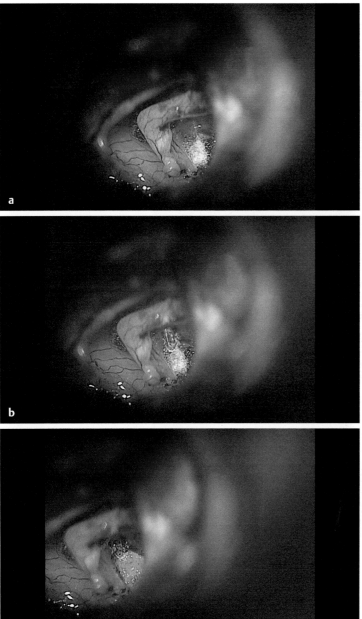

Fig. 33.5 **(a)** The anterior and posterior crura of the stapes. both are seen and could be laserized. **(b)** The anterior crura is laserized. **(c)** The stapes footplate mucosa is decongested by placing gelfoam soaked in adrenaline. *(Continued)*

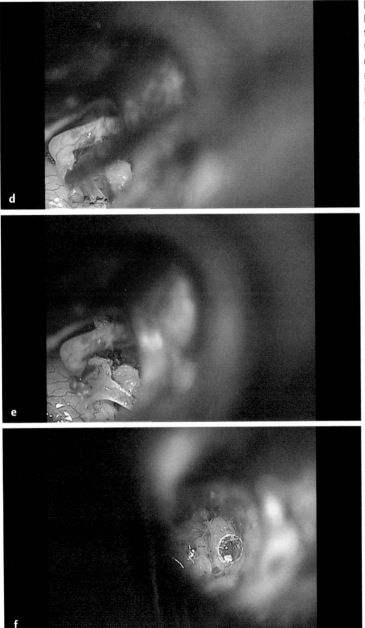

Fig. 33.5 *(Continued)* **(d)** Laserized stapes superstructure is detached from the footplate by a right angle pick. **(e)** The stapes superstructure is removed. **(f)** A fenestra is made in the posterior part of the stapes footplate by CO_2 laser. *(Continued)*

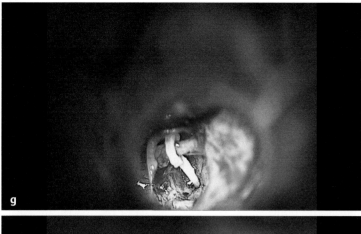

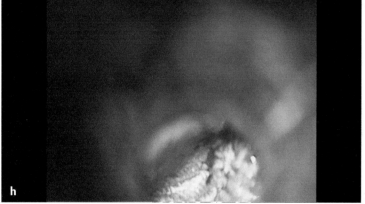

Fig. 33.5 *(Continued)* **(g)** A 0.4-mm piston of suitable length is placed. **(h)** The tympanomeatal (TM) flap is reposited.

Safety of the Facial Nerve to Laser

The bone of the fallopian canal is much thicker than the footplate. Even then, due care should always be taken not to expose the facial nerve to laser beam.

Special care should be taken when the fallopian canal is dehiscent or when the facial nerve is abnormally situated.

Vestibular Safety to Laser

CO_2 laser is very safe for the vestibule.

Laser beam is focused on the lateral surface of the stapes footplate to make a fenestra. Most of its energy is absorbed by the water in the stapes footplate and is used in vaporizing the bone of the stapes footplate to make a discrete fenestra. No laser energy reaches the vestibule. Hence, CO_2 laser is very safe for the vestibule.

Generally, one shot of laser beam is enough to make a discrete fenestra in the stapes footplate and a repeat shot is not required, but when required, there should be a gap of 30 seconds between the two shots to prevent heating of the perilymph.

KTP Laser Stapedotomy

This is a visible laser and is considered not very ideal for stapedotomy. KTP laser is absorbed by colored tissues (red/green) and reflected by white tissue, that is, the bone and cartilage. It is absorbed by blood and hence blood is needed for it to work.

A much higher energy is required in KTP laser than in CO_2 laser to make a fenestra in the stapes footplate. Hence, laser energy passes into the vestibule and can injure the utricle and the saccule.

KTP laser has excellent optical precision but poor tissue interaction.

Disadvantages of using Laser in Stapedectomy

The disadvantages of using laser in stapedectomy are the following:

- Laser assembly is little complicated because the micromanipulator is to be attached to the microscope to which laser is attached. This makes the system little cumbersome, but recent models are less troublesome.

- There is decreased working space between the microscope and the patient's ear because the micromanipulator is projecting beyond the objective lens of the microscope, but this situation can be managed by a microscope with 250-mm objective lens or by using microscope with varioscope.

- Decreased microscope illumination due to the micromanipulator, which is covering the objective lens.

- When CO_2 laser is used, the laser beam and the aiming light beam have to be calibrated frequently to get an accurate effect.

- Both the purchase cost and maintenance cost of the laser tools are high.

Cost of Laser

Both the purchase cost and maintenance cost of the laser tools are high. However, the use of laser in stapes surgery has made the life of the surgeon comfortable. It has also improved results, especially in difficult and complicated situations.

Conclusion

The use of laser in stapes surgery has made the life of the surgeon comfortable. It has also improved surgery results especially in difficult and complicated situations. Many authors using laser have reported excellent results. They also reported very good safety profile with the laser used. Laser stapedectomy to a certain extent reduced technical difficulties of a very technical surgery.

34 Endoscopic Stapes Surgery

Introduction

The endoscope is used not only in stapes surgery but also in other ear surgeries like tympanoplasty, cholesteatoma surgery, and ossiculoplasty.

The advantages of the endoscope over the microscope are the following:

- Wide angle, enabling easy visibility of the stapes and footplate area as compared to the microscope. The anterior crura is also visualized by the endoscope easily, which could never be visualized by the microscope.

- As the footplate area is widely seen by the endoscopes, the need to remove the posterosuperior bony canal wall overhang is less, which has to be removed much more while working with a microscope.

The disadvantages of an endoscopic surgery are the following:

- Lack of depth perception is the biggest disadvantage with the endoscope, especially while doing fine work.

- It is a one-handed surgery. The other hand is occupied in holding the endoscope.

- There is risk of thermal injury to the middle and inner ears from the light source. Thermal injury is more with xenon light than with LED light.

Equipment Used in Endoscopic Surgery

The equipment required for an endoscopic surgery includes a high definition camera with a 14-cm-long rigid endoscope with a diameter of 3 mm, 0 and 30 degrees, along with standard instruments for ear surgery. It is better to have a microdrill and laser along with this (**Fig. 34.1**).

Most of the surgeons use 4-mm, 0- and 30-degree nasal endoscopes for ear surgery, because these are readily available with them and they give a better wide angle view as compared to 3-mm endoscopes.

Surgical Technique

Local anesthesia is preferred for stapedotomy, as a bloodless field is required here. Good hemostasis is needed as one hand of the surgeon is occupied in holding the endoscope and he or she is not able to do repeated suction.

The head end of the operation table should be raised by 15 to 30 degrees to decrease the bleeding. simultaneously, the head should be extended at the neck to get better exposure of the stapes footplate area.

Local anesthesia is injected at the junction of the cartilaginous and bony meatus. One milliliter of 2% lignocaine with 1:200,000 adrenaline is enough.

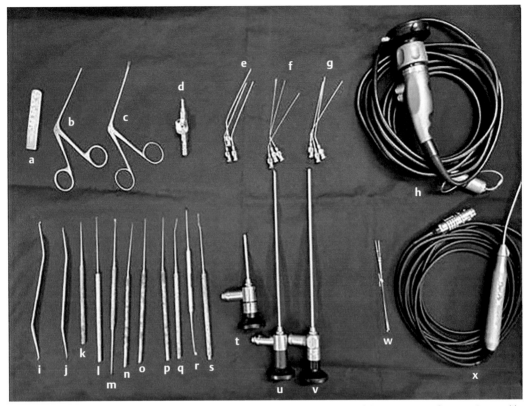

Fig. 34.1   Instrument trolley for endoscopic ear surgery. **(a)** Piston jig. **(b)** Microscopic forceps (crocodile forceps). **(c)** Microscopic scissors. **(d)** Suction adapter. **(e–g)** Suction cannula of different number. **(h)** Endoscopic camera. **(i, j)** Curettes. **(k–r)** Picks, perforators, side knife, and circular knife. **(s)** Distance measuring rod. **(t–v)** Endoscopes. **(w)** Burs. **(x)** Microdrill.

Before starting the surgery, the surgeon should be comfortable with the height of the operation table, with the positioning of the head of the patient, and the height of the monitor.

While using the endoscope, light intensity should be minimum to prevent thermal damage to the middle and inner ear, with intermittent withdrawal of the endoscope for cooling the tissues.

The endoscope provides a wide angle field, magnified view with excellent visualization of the entire middle ear, even in patients with a narrow external auditory canal.

The main problem with endoscopic ear surgery is lack of depth perception, which makes the footplate work more challenging.

The surgical steps in an endoscopic stapes surgery are same as in a microscopic surgery with minor modifications.

Visualization of the entire stapes area including the tympanic part of the facial nerve, handle of the malleus anteriorly and the pyramid posteriorly with the round window inferiorly is achieved without any canal wall removal. even then, some canal wall removal is needed to create more space for easy working in the footplate area, especially in anatomically difficult cases, which makes it easier to place the piston.

Thermal injury to the chorda tympani nerve and the middle ear is prevented by using an LED light source, using minimum intensity of light, and frequent removal of the endoscope for cleaning and defogging. All these reduce the risk of thermal injury by the endoscope.

Other steps are the same as surgery with a microscope. One distinct advantage of performing surgery with an endoscope is its ability to visualize the anterior crus of the stapes and divide it under direct vision. The malleus head fixation can also be addressed with the endoscope with limited atticotomy.

Results

Results of the endoscopic stapes surgery and microscopic stapes surgery were compared in a series of patients, and it was found that postoperative closure of the air–bone gap of up to 10 db was found in around 90% of patients in both groups.

In patients with a narrow external auditory canal, surgery is performed by using a microscope, which requires an endaural incision for getting good exposure. The same patient can be operated on by using an endoscope without endaural incision. That is the advantage of an endoscope over a microscope.

The main problem with the endoscopic ear surgery is lack of depth perception, which makes the footplate work more challenging.

35 Robot-Based Surgery for Otosclerosis

Stapedectomy is the most technical and demanding surgery, and there are a lot of expectations from the surgeon. These expectations of the patient are to be fulfilled by doing a perfect job. During surgery when everything goes right and perfect, you end up with a happy patient with good hearing results and a satisfied surgeon.

If something goes wrong, you will end up with a dizzy and frightened patient. This dizziness takes a lot of time to settle down with decreased hearing or no hearing, which is irreversible (a lifetime trouble). The success rate of surgery is directly proportional to the skill of the surgeon. Now research is going on to use robots for stapes surgery to get better hearing results and less complications following stapedectomy. Robots are designed to provide more accuracy and more stability than human hands, and thus less complications and more success. Various sensors have been designed for navigation, nerve monitoring, force, and chemical sensing. This force sensing plays a very important role while making a fenestra in the stapes footplate by drilling, causing the drill to stop once the fenestra is made. All this research is ongoing and most probably robots are going to be the future of stapes surgery. The robot-based surgery has to prove that it will improve the technique and results of stapes surgery. Complications following robotic surgery should be less compared to the conventional technique.

36 Stapedectomy and Abnormal Facial Nerve

Introduction

When a patient with **progressive** conductive hearing loss with normal tympanic membrane comes to an ENT surgeon, the first diagnosis that they make is otosclerosis, especially in adult patients.

The same thing may not be true in very young patients between the age of 10 and 20 years.

Various causes of significant conductive hearing loss (other than otosclerosis) with normal tympanic membrane in a very young patient are the following:

- Congenital stapedial fixation may be associated with congenital anomaly of the stapes in around 7% of cases.

- Congenital ossicular anomalies may be associated with anomalies of the facial nerve as the embryological development of ossicles, especially the stapes and facial nerve, takes place simultaneously.

These are not the cases of otosclerosis. These are patients with branchial arch anomalies and may be associated with deformity of the external ear and facial asymmetry, which surgeons should always look for before proceeding further.

The associated deafness in these patients is since birth and is nonprogressive.

Various anomalies like slight asymmetry of the face, especially the mandible, and slight deformities of the pinna like a bat ear act as clues for possible congenital middle ear anomalies requiring further investigation like high-resolution computed tomography (HRCT) of the temporal bone (**Figs. 36.1** and **36.2**).

If these minor anomalies of the face and external ear are missed and HRCT scan of temporal bone is not done in these patients, an abnormal middle ear during exploratory tympanotomy in these patients will be a surprise to the surgeon, as he or she never expected this anomaly in the middle ear before starting the surgery.

Regarding the development of the ossicular chain, all these ossicles develop from the first and second branchial arch cartilages.

The head of the malleus and the body of the incus develop from the first arch cartilage.

The handle of the malleus, long process of the incus, and crura of the stapes develop from the second arch cartilage.

The footplate of the stapes develops from the otic capsule.

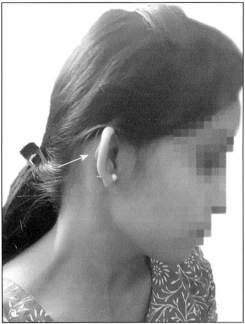
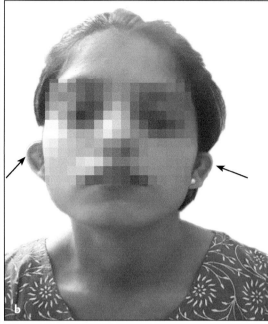

Fig. 36.1 **(a)** A patient with a bat ear (*arrow*). **(b)** A young girl with conductive hearing loss in both ears with normal tympanic membrane having bat ears, *arrows* (branchial arch anomaly). When exploratory tympanotomy was done, anomalies of the facial nerve and ossicular chain were found. Later on, this procedure was abandoned.

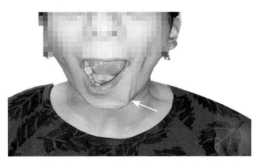

Fig. 36.2 A young girl with conductive hearing loss in both ears with normal tympanic membrane having mandibular asymmetry, *arrow* (branchial arch anomaly). When exploratory tympanotomy was done, anomalies of the facial nerve and the ossicular chain were found. Later on, this procedure was abandoned.

There are three types of anomalies of the facial nerve in relation to the oval window:

1. Dehiscent fallopian canal and an overhanging (prolapsed) facial nerve (commonest). This prolapse may be partial or complete.

2. A facial nerve coursing over the promontory.

3. A bifid facial nerve (rare).

These are nothing but anomalies of the first and second branchial arches and are associated with various anomalies in the middle ear structures, especially the ossicles.

Classification of the Ossicular Anomalies

Ossicular anomalies could be classified into the following:

- Class 1: Stapedial fixation.

- Class 2: Stapedial fixation with other ossicular anomaly.

- Class 3: Other ossicular anomaly. No stapedial fixation.

- Class 4: Oval window/round window dysplasia.

These anomalies are associated with numerous syndromes. For example, the Klippel–Feil syndrome in which there are anomalies of the incus and stapes with incudostapedial (IS) joint deformity.

Investigations

As already mentioned, doubt about the possibility of getting facial nerve anomalies during stapedectomy usually occurs in a very young patient with conductive hearing loss with facial asymmetry, especially the mandibular asymmetry.

In these cases, preoperative HRCT scan of the temporal bone gives an idea about the difficult situations, and their systematic use helps in obtaining better postoperative results.

The commonest facial nerve anomaly is the dehiscent fallopian canal with a prolapsed facial nerve. This prolapsed facial nerve touches the stapes superstructure as shown in **Fig. 36.3**.

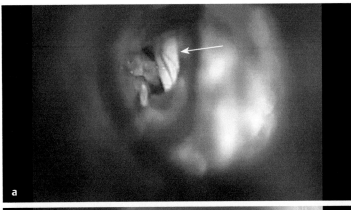

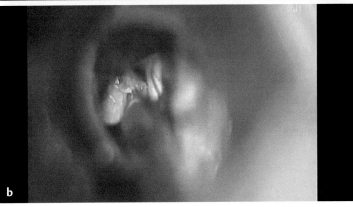

Fig. 36.3 (a) A dehiscent facial nerve touching the stapes superstructure (*arrow*). **(b)** The stapes superstructure drilled carefully by a microdrill and removed. *(Continued)*

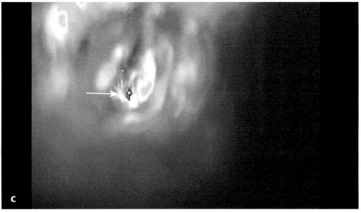

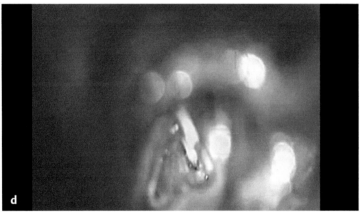

Fig. 36.3 *(Continued)* **(c)** After removal of stapes super-structure, the footplate of the stapes is seen. A fenestra *(arrow)* is made in the posterior part of the footplate by a microdrill. Laser is not used here. **(d)** A Teflon piston of suitable length and 0.4 mm thickness is placed and tightened. The tympanomeatal flap is reposited.

Various ossicular anomalies like absent or malformed stapes, absent oval window, malformed incus, facial nerve coursing over the promontory, and bifid facial nerve are shown in **Fig. 36.4**.

Bifid Facial Nerve with Stapes in Between

The bifid facial nerve with fixed stapes in between is depicted in **Fig. 36.5a**. The stape-dotomy was performed using a microdrill (**Fig. 36.5b**). Laser was not used. A fenestra of 0.6 mm was made by using diamond bur (**Fig. 36.5c**) and 0.4-mm piston of suitable length was placed and tightened, and the tympanomeatal (TM) flap was reposited (**Fig. 36.5d**).

Conclusion

A very young patient with conductive hearing loss with normal tympanic membrane is not necessary a patient of otosclerosis.

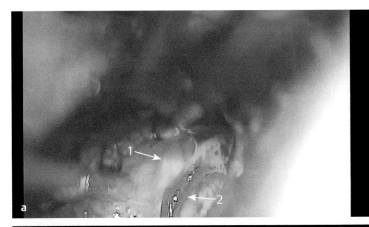

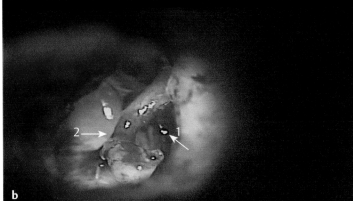

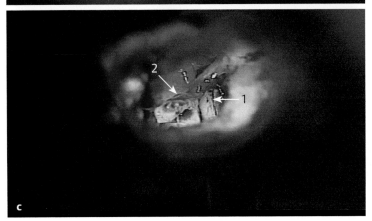

Fig. 36.4 **(a)** A big naked facial nerve running horizontally over the promontory (as shown by *arrow* 1). No oval window, no stapes, malformed incus (*arrow 2*), and normal malleus. **(b)** Abnormal ossicular chain, no oval window, no stapes, facial nerve at the level of the oval window (*arrow 1*), abnormal incus with remnants of the head and the crura of the stapes (*arrow 2*), and normal malleus. **(c)** Abnormal ossicular chain, no oval window, no stapes, facial nerve at the level of the oval window (*arrow 1*), abnormal incus (*arrow 2*), normal malleus. *(Continued)*

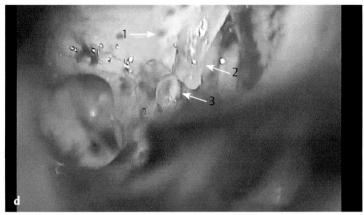

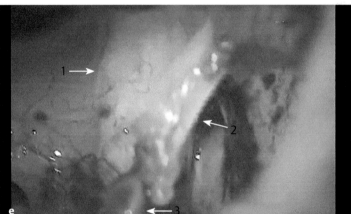

Fig. 36.4 *(Continued)* **(d)** A big naked facial nerve running horizontally over the promontory *(arrow 1)*, no oval window, malformed incus *(arrow 2)*, and rudimentary stapes head and crura *(arrow 3)*, but no footplate. **(e)** A big naked facial nerve running horizontally over the promontory *(arrow 1)*, no oval window, malformed incus *(arrow 2)*, and rudimentary stapes head and crura *(arrow 3)* but no footplate (under higher magnification).

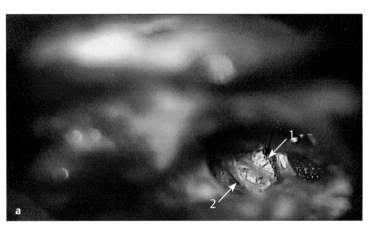

Fig. 36.5 **(a)** A bifid facial nerve *(arrows 1 and 2)* with the stapes footplate in between. The stapes superstructure has been removed. *(Continued)*

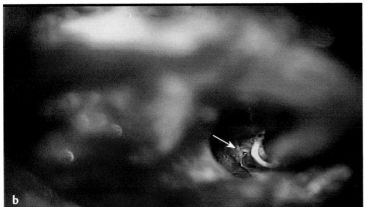

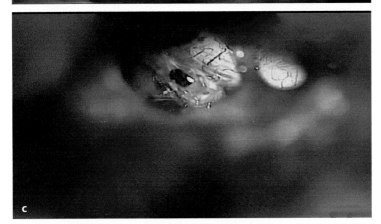

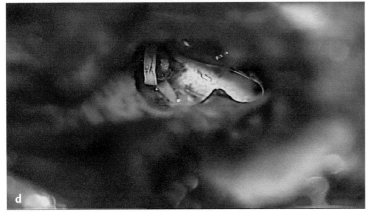

Fig. 36.5 *(Continued)* **(b)** A bifid facial nerve with the stapes footplate in between (*arrow*). A fenestra is made by a microdrill. **(c)** A bifid facial nerve. A 0.6-mm fenestra is made in the footplate by a microdrill using a 0.6-mm diamond bur. **(d)** A Teflon piston of suitable length and 0.4 mm thickness is placed and tightened, and the tympanomeatal (TM) flap is reposited.

The possibility of other congenital ossicular and facial nerve anomalies should always be considered in a very young patient with conductive hearing loss having normal tympanic membrane.

Always look for any associated facial asymmetry, especially mandibular asymmetry.

HRCT scan of the temporal bone should always be done in these patients to decide further action, so that proper treatment can be carried out.

37 Stapedotomy in Children

It is most important to diagnose the cause of conductive deafness in young children. The first thing is to rule out eustachian tube (ET) dysfunction with serous otitis media, which can be diagnosed by clinical examination as well as by impedance audiogram.

When there is no serous otitis media and ET dysfunction, two main causes of conductive deafness are found in children especially when the tympanic membrane is normal:

Congenital fixation of the stapes footplate: The deafness in these patients is since birth and by the time they realize deafness, they are between the age of 10 and 12 years. Usually, there is no family history.

The deafness in these patients is nonprogressive. Usually, there is no tinnitus. If the disease is bilateral, which is rare, speech is affected. The air–bone (AB) gap in these patients is more as compared to otosclerosis. Around 45 to 55 dB conductive hearing loss is found at all the frequencies.

Computed tomography (CT) scan of the temporal bone should always be done in these patients not only to confirm the diagnosis but also to rule out any associated anomalies of the malleus, incus, and inner ear, especially the cochlear aqueduct.

There is total fixation of stapes footplate here. its margin and annular ligament cannot be distinguished easily.

Surgery in these patients is risky due to the high possibility of perilymph gusher.

Otosclerosis: The diagnosis is confirmed by ruling out other causes of conductive hearing loss by clinical examination, pure tone audiogram, impedance audiogram, and high-resolution CT (HRCT) of the temporal bone. Audiogram shows conductive hearing loss mainly in low frequency. Most times, a family history of otosclerosis is present.

Stapedectomy is the treatment. Surgery is the same as in adults, and long-term results are equally good.

Surgery results are good and remain good if proper care is taken to avoid upper respiratory tract infection (URI). If the child gets URI, that should be treated promptly.

If there are adenoids, they should be taken care of before stapedectomy.

Young children are always very active. After stapedectomy, they should avoid certain sports where there is a possibility of head trauma. Football, boxing, and wrestling should be avoided after stapedectomy in children.

38 Stapedotomy Following Tympanoplasty

Patients having perforated ear drum with stapes fixation, confirmed by gelfoam patch test, should be subjected to first-stage tympanoplasty.

Tympanoplasty and stapedotomy cannot be performed together, because the inner ear cannot be opened unless the tympanic membrane is intact.

Hearing improvement in patients in which stapedotomy has been performed after tympanoplasty is less as compared to patients with pure otosclerosis.

The results of surgery in these patients are not as good as in patients with otosclerosis without otitis media.

In these patients the air-bone gap after stapedectomy is more as compared to patients with pure otosclerosis.

The cause for this comparative poor results in these patients is the associated effect of otitis media on the overall mobility of the ossicular chain and some blunting of the tympanic membrane following myringoplasty, but even then, the results are quite satisfactory and patients are quite happy. Hence, stapedotomy should always be performed after tympanoplasty if required.

The stapedial fixation associated with otitis media is due to either otosclerosis or tympanosclerosis. The long-term hearing results of stapedotomy are better in otosclerotic patients than in tympanosclerotic patients.

Index